HEALING WITH NUTRITIONAL THERAPY

GW00802265

This series introduces a wide range of healing techniques that can be used either independently or as a complement to traditional medical treatment. Most of the techniques included in the series can be learnt and practised alone, and each encourages a degree of self-reliance, offering the tools needed to achieve and maintain an optimum state of health.

Each title opens with information on the history and principles of the technique and goes on to offer practical and straightforward guidance on ways in which it can be applied, with diagrams and case studies where appropriate. Please note that readers are advised to seek professional guidance for serious ailments, and to make use of the list of practitioners for further guidance. Many of the techniques in this series are taught in workshops and adult education classes; all of the titles are written by professional practitioners with many years of experience and proven track records.

AVAILABLE IN THIS SERIES

Healing with Ayurveda — Angela Hope-Murray and
    Tony Pickup

Healing with Colour — Helen Graham

Healing with Crystals — Jacquie Burgess

Healing with Essential Oils — Nicola Naylor

Healing with Herbs — Judith Hoad

Healing with Homeopathy — Peter Chappell and
    David Andrews

Healing with Meditation — Doriel Hall

Healing with Osteopathy — Peta Sneddon and Paolo Coseschi

Healing with Reflexology — Rosalind Oxenford

Healing with Shiatsu — Catherine Sutton

Healing with Nutritional Therapy

PATRICIA QUINN

Newleaf

Newleaf

an imprint of
Gill & Macmillan Ltd
Hume Avenue, Park West
Dublin 12
with associated companies throughout the world
www.gillmacmillan.ie
© Patricia Quinn 1998
0 7171 2626 9
Series editor: Tessa Strickland
Series copy editor: Pamela Dix
Index compiled by Helen Litton
Original text design by Identikit Design Consultants, Dublin
Print origination by Carole Lynch
Printed by ColourBooks Ltd, Dublin

This book is typeset in 10/15 pt Bembo.

The paper used in this book comes from the wood pulp of
managed forests. For every tree felled, at least one tree is planted,
thereby renewing natural resources.

A catalogue record is available for this book from
the British Library.

3 5 7 6 4

Contents

CHAPTER ONE

What is Nutritional Therapy?

Nutritional therapy is a system of healing based on the belief that food as nature intended provides the medicine we need to obtain and maintain a state of health: our food is our medicine and our medicine is our food. Although some health problems require specific medication, many conditions can be relieved effectively with nutritional therapy. This includes disorders ranging from chronic fatigue, energy loss, insomnia and depression to back ache, skin complaints, asthma and headaches. Nutritional therapy will also benefit you if you have no specific illness, but want to maintain a state of optimum health. It is safe for babies and children as well as adults, and the change of eating patterns that is typically prescribed usually has far fewer side effects than many synthetic medicines.

Nutritional therapy is a holistic discipline; nutrition as the key to good health is the all-embracing fundamental principle which has been used since the time of the famous Greek doctor and founder of western medicine, Hippocrates, to help people of all ages to stay at their personal peak of energy and vitality. Today, the new insights of food scientists play a significant role in the practice of nutritional therapy as preventative medicine.

During the last fifty years, there have been many wonderful breakthroughs in our understanding of the role of food in our lives. But at the same time, it is becoming apparent to many of us that food is the cornerstone which, in our modern lifestyle, has been rejected by the builder.

The very speed at which we live and work — the pressure of the deadline — pushes us into a fast-eating culture, where quality of food becomes secondary. Eating on the job, on the run, under pressure, denies us the experience, the purpose and the role of food. Eventually it denies us even our very lifestyle. Modern supermarkets are stocked with many instant meals, but more often than not, these meals are far lower in nutritional value than those prepared at home with fresh, organically grown ingredients.

For all the benefits that agribusiness has brought the people of the western world, the disadvantages of the modern food industry include extensive use of chemicals in food production. There is also a loss of the vitality that is intrinsic in newly harvested food, due to many products being transported vast distances before they reach their destination. Of course, this is the case with many of the so-called 'fresh' foods on our supermarket shelves, let alone those dishes that have been pre-cooked and packaged before reaching the supermarkets.

Lifestyle and nutrition are intimately linked, and our lifestyle defines itself partly from the tradition of the country we live in and partly from our attitudes. How do you really want to live? Given the choice, would you prefer to eat well every day, to exercise, to breathe good, clean air as often as possible, to take a reasonable amount of water in order to keep your bloodstream clean and able to wash out toxins? This choice is available to all of us, but to exercise that choice we need to understand the impact on our well-being of different foods and learn from direct experience what kind of eating pattern best suits our lifestyle.

WHAT IS HEALTH?

In a dynamic and good state of health, the mental, emotional, physical and spiritual entities all live in harmony with each other. For a wider comprehension of health, it is interesting to look at the issue of 'healthiness' not only from the western but also from the eastern viewpoint.

The ancient systems of Chinese and Indian medicine go back more than 5,000 years. These cultures used — and continue to use — whole plants in their treatment, whereas orthodox medicine uses extracts from plants; these extracts are often then replicated by synthetic products.

The two systems of medicine diverge at the point of prevention. Eastern practices include the preventative care of the whole person as a primary aim — to maintain good health. The formula for good health is:

- life force
- good-quality blood
- proper nourishment.

Our daily diet will make good-quality blood; healthy energy flows in a body with such good blood. We need to ask ourselves daily questions. What is my physical health like today? Do I have a sense of well-being? Have I got plenty of energy? Do I sleep and eat well? How we feel each day is built upon our past actions, our past dietary practices, whether we have taken physical exercise, whether we have been mentally active and our general attitude towards life.

TIREDNESS VERSUS FATIGUE

Fatigue is very prevalent in the present day. The healthy person who uses his or her entire body in the ways described above during each day will feel tired — the pleasant feeling of having worked hard. This individual's body will be able to relax completely and recuperate at the end of the day. This is not fatigue — it is the body's natural need for rest. It is during rest and recuperation that the body cleanses itself of all the toxins which build up during activity. If the body is not given a chance to self-cleanse, a state of fatigue will become persistent. When it becomes chronic, fatigue may indicate underlying problems, such as infection, immune system weaknesses, glandular problems or lymphatic congestion, as the body's systems become clogged by waste.

WHAT IS ILLNESS?

Illness develops in four stages:
- tiredness, changing to fatigue — no amount of rest seems adequate
- irritability
- symptoms
- illness.

The oriental approach to health divides the causes of illness into two: those which come from within, and those which come from without. Those from within are mostly to do with our lifestyle, our traditions and our beliefs. The ways in which we can be affected from within are as follows:
- excess of even positive emotions, such as joy, can affect the heart
- excess of anger can affect the liver
- excess of sadness damages the appetite, the stomach, spleen or pancreas
- excessive grief can affect the lungs
- shock, fear, surprise or fright can affect the kidneys.

Part of the process of nutritional therapy is to help us to restore the proper balance, to bring about the harmony that we are lacking.

THE 'FOUR DOCTORS'

The basic needs of our physical bodies to eliminate toxic waste, as described above, are being denied to us by the life we lead in modern western society. What we require to cater for these basic needs I call the 'four doctors':

1 sunlight and fresh air
2 proper exercise and sufficient rest
3 good food
4 pure water.

While our ancestors lived mainly outdoor lives, we tend to live largely indoors, denying ourselves the most pivotal requirement: light. Our whole body depends upon the reception of light in order to carry out vital functions — the regulation of the appetite, our patterns of sleeping and waking, aspects of our behaviour and the health of our nervous system. Fresh air is necessary so that we may exchange the toxins and pollutants in the body with at least an equal amount of air. Otherwise, we develop acute respiratory problems due to overload; our cities do not have sufficient trees to breathe back oxygen into our environment. Trees act as 'lungs', by filling the air with life-giving oxygen.

Water is the greatest treat for the body. It is the river which carries all the nutrients around the body to the brain, and to every single cell in the body. The brain is the first place to suffer dehydration — it then becomes very difficult to think, or to make appropriate decisions. In recent studies of long-distance walkers, it was found that water helped more than food to give them the energy to finish. Likewise, those driving for long distances need not only a break of fifteen minutes or so, but also a snack, in order to maintain their concentration on the road. In both of these examples, the simple remedies given prevented emotional and psychological imbalance, which drains the body of its energy supply and causes fatigue.

THE ROLE OF FOOD IN OUR LIVES

By experimenting with the effects of different foods, many people find that they also revise old beliefs and ideas about the role of food in their lives. Nutritional therapy is not just about eating different types of food; it is also about increasing your awareness of how you eat and also of where the food you eat comes from, how you store and prepare it, and how you perceive yourself and your place in the web of life. The benefits of nutritional therapy are sometimes immediate, but its study is timeless and its effects can bring about long-lasting changes in your attitude to life.

Recently, Dr Henry Dreher — author of *The Immune Power Personality* — reminded us of certain characteristics which we can all develop, and which increase our ability to be healthy. These characteristics include:

- having the ability to recognise when the body is signalling to us that it is in pain, or feeling tired
- identifying emotions such as anger or sadness
- connecting these states to food that we have recently eaten and so learning to identify the effects that different foods have on us
- developing a sense of control over our health and over the quality of our lives, because the way we live — as well as the way we eat — is part of the way we nourish ourselves.

Nutritional therapy helps us to consider our human immunity in the context of a rapidly changing environment, by deepening our understanding of the dynamic ebb and flow between ourselves and our outer world, which is going on at all times. Our immunity is part of the entire picture — a relationship between our own evolving and our world. 'Whole body' immunity concerns all aspects of life: ensuring that the physical body has the correct nutrition and appropriate healing therapies; enjoying good emotional health by nurturing the feelings; learning to make choices from a position of unbiased awareness and not from the 'victim' or 'martyr' approach.

Nutritional therapy requires us to acknowledge that we are body, soul, mind and emotion. Accordingly, it incorporates all these aspects of our lives, with the objective that we maintain a healthy mind and soul as well as a healthy body; develop an open-minded outlook and a positive attitude to ourselves; and learn to see any causes of stress in our lives as challenges rather than threats.

CHAPTER TWO

The History of Nutritional Healing

A monk asked, 'Is there anything more miraculous than the wonders of Nature?' The master replied, 'Yes — your appreciation of the wonders of Nature.'

In Ancient Greece, the two philosophies of medicine and healing were under the patronage of two different gods. The doctors worked under the patronage of Asklepios, god of medicine, while Asklepios's beautiful daughter Hygeia (goddess of health, whose name is the origin of the word 'hygiene') was the patron of healers. In around 400 BC, Hippocrates was writing his memoirs on the medicinal uses of herbs, spices and food. At about the same time, and of equal importance, the man known as the father of botany, Theophrastus, was recording the extensive botanical knowledge of the day, and the wide variety of uses which herbs and spices were found to have.

Later, when the Romans occupied Britain in the first century AD, they looked after the medical needs of their soldiers with a variety of herbs and spices. In fact, they brought 400 herbs with them to Britain, which they planted and harvested. These new herbs added to an already extensive body of knowledge that had been handed down from generation to generation by the druids — herbs are an ancient part of Europe's heritage.

In the sixth century, after the Dark Ages, the religious orders began to found their monasteries. They grew their herbs in kitchen gardens, while the hospitals filled their gardens with herbs with which to feed the sick. Spices were, of course, as highly prized as gold, because they were so difficult to get from the Orient and the near east.

There was a widely held traditional belief among the ordinary people, who in their own kitchens were cooking vegetables, grains, fruit and meats, that these spices also held the elements necessary to heal disease.

JAMES LIND'S CURE FOR SCURVY

In the year 1747, James Lind, who was the surgeon's mate on the HMS *Salisbury*, made the brilliant discovery that two oranges and one lemon eaten daily over a six-day period completely reversed the symptoms of scurvy (a vitamin C deficiency, which caused widespread weakness, disease and death among sailors). Lind did not know anything about vitamins, but his remedy was extremely effective. He had used food as medicine. Yet it was only in 1795 that the British admiralty put his simple, preventative medicine into action. From 1795, an ounce of lemon juice per day wiped out scurvy in the English Merchant Navy. Many more years were to pass, however, before this simple preventative measure was extended to the Royal Navy.

THE EFFECTS OF REFINED FOODS

During the early nineteenth century, further experiments with food proved that the fat, carbohydrate and protein content of food — while essential for life — were not sufficient to support growth, nor for the healthy development of the eyes. When Mullen in Switzerland built the steel roller mill in 1830, white flour became cheaper and more widely available. Until then, the people of Europe had eaten a wide variety of fruits, vegetables, grains, herbs and, latterly, spices. The change in diet to refined white flour, white rice and white sugar caused widespread vitamin deficiency. Serious illnesses such as beriberi became known wherever these foods spread.

In the West Indies, a young Dutch physician called
Christiaan Eijkman was assigned in 1886 to study beriberi.
He observed that the chickens in the laboratory chicken
yard were suffering from a disease which paralleled all the
symptoms of beriberi. He discovered through a process of
observation and enquiry that the regular diet of the
patients in the military hospital was white rice. Most of
the chickens were fed the leftovers, but when a new cook
took over, he refused to feed the patients anything other
than whole grain, unpolished rice. With this change, both
the patients and the chickens revived and went on to
become very healthy.

Eijkman then did an enormous study of Dutch
West Indies prisoners. He found that beriberi was 300
times more prevalent in prisoners where polished (white)
rice rather than unpolished rice was the staple diet.
He concluded that the bran of the rice contained a
substance, or nutrient, necessary for health.

NATUROPATHIC MEDICINE

Right up to the present day, the debate continues about
the very nature of health. But the most basic tenet of all
healing — whether it be mental, emotional, physical,
spiritual, chemical, or all these things — is that nature
heals. This was the central theme of naturopathic
medicine, which was the precursor to nutritional
therapy.

A great surge in natural therapies occurred in the
nineteenth century in Europe and America, and written
legacies of enormous value were produced by naturopaths
such as Vincent Priessnitz, Jethro Kloss, Sebastian Kneipp
and J. H. Kellogg. While some physicians chose to
specialise in naturopathic medicine, others — throughout

the world — worked within their own sphere of
medicine, developing, expanding and increasing their
understanding of nutrition within the context of a
particular discipline. While working with the principles
that outside intervention is necessary on the one hand,
and that nature works towards healing on the other, the
naturopath's approach maintains that the constant effort
of the body's life force is always in the direction of self-
cleansing, self-repair and positive health. According to this
approach, every cell in the body is imbued with an instinct
of self-preservation, which is sustained by an inherent
force known as 'the vital force of life'.

THE DISCOVERY OF VITAMINS

In 1911, the Polish scientist Casimir Funk proposed the
theory that there were anti-scurvy, anti-beriberi, anti-
pellagra and anti-rickets factors in food. He called these
food factors 'vitamins' (from the Latin *vita*, meaning
'life'). Then, Albert Szent-Györgyi of Budapest gave the
crystalline substance he had isolated from the adrenal
gland of the ox to the English sugar chemist W. N.
Haworth, who found its structural formula. It was
ascorbic acid — the acidic substance which prevents
scurvy! In 1937, these two men each received a Nobel
prize for their great work in finally finding the substance
which in 1747 James Lind had proven, through a simple
test with oranges and lemons, to save people's lives at sea.
Extensive research into vitamins in subsequent decades
has established that we need a balanced intake of vitamins
A, B, C, D and E to maintain health. Lists of foods
containing these vitamins are included in Appendix One
(see pages 101–2).

THE DISCOVERY OF MINERALS

The study of minerals in food began in the 1940s — until that time, only iodine and iron were known and understood to be essential to life. Since the 1940s, numerous major discoveries have been made — we now know of a whole range of minerals which are essential to good health, such as zinc, iodine and potassium. By identifying vitamin and mineral imbalances, today's doctors can reverse many serious illnesses that were previously undiagnosable.

THE BIRTH OF NUTRITIONAL MEDICINE

In 1968, Dr Linus Pauling defined orthomolecular medicine, with particular reference to psychiatry as a way of achieving and preserving mental health by varying the concentrations in the human body of substances that are normally present, such as vitamins. This definition was the crystallisation of what we now know as nutritional medicine. Dr Pauling won the Nobel Prize for Chemistry in 1954, and the Nobel Prize for Peace in 1963. His pioneering work gave medicine a new impetus. Until his research was recognised, nutrition and medicine had become polarised as separate professions.

In recent decades, a succession of nutritional breakthroughs all over the world has gradually brought new evidence to light about the properties in food that are essential to good health. The Hippocratic school, which treated disease with diet, fasting, hydrotherapy, exercise and spinal manipulation, may yet become recognised once more as a cornerstone of medical practice.

LOCAL FOOD

The gastronomic life of a country used to be based primarily on climate and geographical position, so this suggests that there may have been some uniformity in eating patterns among people who live along particular latitudes and in similar land-masses. But occupation by peoples with other eating habits can radically affect the native diet. This is how viniculture superseded beer and apple brewing in Europe, following the Roman occupation of England and France. But national preferences for foods die hard, because they are deeply associated with the culture — not just the dinner plate.

THE IMPACT OF INDUSTRIALISATION ON DIET

The impact of industrialisation, however, particularly in the sphere of agriculture, and the new wave of technology, have contributed to a loss of awareness about our local dietary heritage. In England, the movement from a rural and agricultural society to an urban, industrial society in the nineteenth century had devastating effects on workers' diets. Widespread malnutrition was dealt with at that time through the mass production and distribution of basic foodstuffs by religious institutions, in particular the Quaker foundations and families such as Fry and Cadbury. The era of processed food was about to dawn. And it was the answer to a definite demand.

At first, this kind of food relieved malnutrition and susceptibility to contagious diseases, so how is it today that processed food adds to our health problems? That processed food is directly linked with obesity, diabetes, heart disease and cancer is irrefutable. But there are many additional contributing factors. For example, most of us take far less exercise than we did in the centuries before the invention of the car; prior to the revolution in transport and technology, the pace of life was far slower than it is now; and before the introduction of intensive farming techniques, processed foods were typically combined with locally grown produce.

Nutritional analysts have observed that when a country industrialises slowly, its people have maintained their cultural heritage in general and their food heritage in particular. Southern France, Italy and Spain, the coast of the Middle East and the islands all share the now revered 'Mediterranean Diet'. They still adhere to their regional preferences, but have in common with other coast-dwelling peoples such as the Scandinavians and Japanese access to certain very beneficial sea foods. By comparison, the people of countries which have industrialised rapidly, such as England and, more recently, Japan (where these changes are beginning to make detrimental inroads on the benefits of the traditional diet) and parts of China, rapidly lose touch with their food heritage. Time becomes a precious commodity, and as fewer people work on the land, knowledge of the qualities in local food diminishes, while less nutritious, imported food products become fashionable. For example, processed cereals are now a feature of most English households, yet these are both more expensive and less nutritious than a simple dish such as porridge with dried fruits. Similarly, in many parts of Japan, refined white bread has replaced a more nutritious traditional breakfast of egg, rice and bean curd.

THE EFFECTS OF INTENSIVE AGRICULTURE
Overall, we can see that while research into the nutrients of food has made a huge contribution to our knowledge during the course of the twentieth century, at the same time loss of local knowledge — combined with intensive use of artificial fertilisers in food cultivation and the export

of basic foodstuffs on a massive scale — have contributed to a deterioration in our overall health. However, once you understand the central significance of food in your life, you can make several quite simple adjustments to your eating patterns to ensure that you receive the nutrients you need. You do not have to be a chemist or a scientist to benefit from the insights of nutritional therapy; the next section of this book will show how many of the precepts of nutritional therapy are based on simple self-awareness, self-observation and common sense.

CHAPTER THREE

Essential Nutrients

The body requires a certain daily intake of nutrients in the form of carbohydrates, fats, minerals, proteins, vitamins and water. If your body is deficient in any of these, illness will be the result. Sometimes the illness may be due to a clear absence of the appropriate nutrient in your diet; in other instances, the deficiency may arise because of the body's inability to absorb a particular nutrient properly. In these cases, an alternative way of providing that nutrient needs to be found.

CARBOHYDRATES

Carbohydrates are the body's major source of energy, and are made up of sugars, starch and fibre. They are also needed to metabolise proteins for body tissue repair, and to run the central nervous system. Unrefined carbohydrates include all grains, such as rice, wheat, oats, barley and millet. They lose their nutritional value through refinement and provide only 'empty' calories (e.g. white bread, white rice and white sugar).

Lack of carbohydrates leads to listlessness, fatigue and nausea. Too many refined carbohydrates lead to obesity, tooth decay, high blood pressure, heart disease and diabetes.

FATS

Fats are needed for energy and to create layers of protective tissue in the body. They provide over twice as much energy, weight for weight, as carbohydrates and proteins. So comparatively little fat is needed in the average diet.

Fats are divided into three categories: saturated, monounsaturated and polyunsaturated. Saturated fats are found mainly in food from animal sources, including full-fat milk, cheese, eggs, cream and butter. These saturated fats also contain high amounts of cholesterol.

Monounsaturated and polyunsaturated fats are found mainly in vegetable oils and soft margarines. They contain no cholesterol. Polyunsaturated fats also contain three essential acids: linoleic acid, oleic acid and arachidonic acid. Linoleic acid enables the body to synthesise other fats from food. It is also thought to help reduce the level of cholesterol in the blood.

Too much fat can lead to obesity, which increases the risk of diabetes, high blood pressure, arthritis and gall-bladder disease.

FOLIC ACID

Folic acid is one of the B vitamins (see below). It helps in the formation of RNA and DNA, and in the breakdown of proteins into amino acids. It is especially important in the early months of pregnancy. Lack of folic acid leads to poor growth, to gastrointestinal problems and to anaemia.

MINERALS

Minerals are vital for cell growth and repair and the self-regulation of the body. The macro-minerals (calcium, phosphorus, magnesium, sodium, potassium and chloride) are needed in quantities of 100 mg or more per day. The micro-minerals (iron, iodine and zinc) are needed in far smaller quantities. A balance of minerals is very important, as they often work in conjunction with each other.

CALCIUM

Calcium is essential for the healthy growth of bones, teeth, nails and hair, for the functioning of the nervous system, and for maintenance of muscular contractions. It is present in almonds, almond spreads, fish, molasses, sunflower seeds, sunflower seed spread, green vegetables, kelp, sea vegetables such as kombu, wakame, dulse, and hiziki, sesame seeds, tahini (sesame spread), tofu, cottage cheese, cheddar cheese, goat's milk, cheese and yoghurt, sheep's milk, cheese and feta cheese, ricotta cheese and natural yoghurt. Lack of calcium can lead to muscular problems, brittle bones and tooth decay. It can also cause insomnia and nervous exhaustion.

CHLORIDE

Chloride is needed with sodium and potassium to regulate the body's fluids. It helps in the formation of gastric juices in the stomach for the effective digestion of proteins. Lack of chloride can lead to an imbalance of sodium in the body.

IODINE

Iodine is necessary for the formation and healthy functioning of two hormones in the thyroid gland which regulate metabolism and protein synthesis. Lack of iodine can lead to obesity, swelling and listlessness.

IRON

Iron is necessary for the formation of haemoglobin red blood cells, which transport oxygen from the lungs all round the body. To work effectively, iron needs to be balanced with a trace of copper and vitamin C. Lack of iron leads to anaemia and fatigue.

MAGNESIUM

Magnesium combines with calcium and phosphorus for the healthy functioning of the skeletal and nervous systems. Lack of magnesium causes muscular weakness and delirium.

PHOSPHORUS

Phosphorus combines with calcium for the healthy formation of bones and teeth, and assists in the body's release of energy.

POTASSIUM

Potassium works with sodium to regulate the body's fluids, particularly in the muscle cells and the blood. Lack of potassium can lead to impaired neuromuscular functioning and even to heart attacks.

SODIUM

Sodium regulates the body's fluid balance and monitors the passage of nutrients into, and waste out of, the cells. Too much sodium causes fluid retention and high blood pressure.

SULPHUR

Sulphur constitutes 0.05 per cent of the earth's crust. It is a constituent of all proteins and is present in a number of amino acids. It is also found in vitamin D, thiamine and biotin. It is present in the nails, skin, joints and hair. Sulphur can be obtained from a wide range of sources, some of which include eggs, nuts, garlic, poultry, meat, fish, milk, cheese, mustard and cress, pears, apricots and oatmeal.

ZINC

Zinc is essential for the growth and repair of tissues, for protein synthesis and for the body's immune system. Lack of zinc causes fatigue, low resistance to infection and stunted sexual maturity.

PROTEINS

Proteins are essential for the formation, growth and repair of all body cells, and for the functioning of the enzymes, hormones and antibodies which regulate and control our bodies. Proteins are made up of amino acids. There are about twenty amino acids, eight of which are present in protein-containing foods. The rest are synthesised by the body from these eight. Foods which contain all of the eight essential amino acids are called complete, or first-class, proteins; foods which contain only a few are referred to as incomplete, or second-class, proteins.

Dairy products, meat, eggs and fish all contain first-class protein. Vegetable proteins such as peas, beans and lentils, grains and vegetables are called second-class proteins, because they do not contain the full spectrum of essential building blocks, or essential amino acids. However, many traditional peoples combine second-class, non-meat foods in a way which comfortably fulfils our minds' and bodies' protein requirements, without the detrimental effects that can accompany a meat-rich diet. In 1971, the American food writer Frances Moore Lappé introduced the idea of complementary proteins to modern readers with her book *Diet for a Small Planet*, which is now regarded as a classic and has been translated into many languages.

Lack of protein leads to a decrease in the metabolic process and, in extreme cases of deprivation, eventually to starvation.

VITAMINS

Vitamins are usually needed only in tiny quantities, but
they are crucial to the healthy functioning of the body.
Vitamins are classified in six groups: A, B, C, D, E and K.
Vitamins in groups B and C are water-soluble, which
means they must be taken regularly as the body cannot
store them for a long period of time; vitamins in groups
A, D, E and K are fat-soluble and so last rather longer.

VITAMIN A (RETINOL)

Vitamin A helps in cell differentiation. It is also needed for
healthy skin and mucous membranes and for good night
vision. Lack of vitamin A leads to softening of the bones
and teeth, dry skin and night blindness.

VITAMIN B

The major function of the B vitamins is to break down
food into simple sugar molecules for energy and to form
new red blood cells. The B vitamins are also important
for the healthy functioning of the brain, nervous and
circulatory systems, and for healthy hair, skin and eyes.
B vitamins work most effectively in conjunction with
each other.

VITAMIN B1 (THIAMINE)

Vitamin B1 breaks down carbohydrates for energy. It also
assists the functioning of the brain, nerves and muscles.
Lack of vitamin B1 leads to constipation and abdominal
pains, and in extreme cases to beriberi.

VITAMIN B2 (RIBOFLAVIN)

Vitamin B2 breaks down fats, carbohydrates and proteins
for energy. It is easily destroyed by exposure to light. Lack

of vitamin B2 leads to mouth and throat infections and eye fatigue. Riboflavin deficiency is common in non-milk drinkers.

VITAMIN B3 (NIACIN)

Vitamin B3 breaks down fats, carbohydrates and proteins for energy. Lack of vitamin B3 leads to digestive disorders, a sore, swollen tongue and impairment of growth in children.

VITAMIN B6 (PYRIDOXINE)

Vitamin B6 breaks down proteins into amino acids for the formation of red blood cells and hormones. Lack of vitamin B6 leads to anaemia, nervous disorders and fatigue.

VITAMIN B12 (COBALAMIN)

Vitamin B12 is essential for the formation of red blood cells and for synthesising RNA and DNA. It is also essential for the healthy functioning of the nervous system. Dairy products are a rich source of vitamin B12. Lack of vitamin B12 leads to serious anaemia.

VITAMIN C (ASCORBIC ACID)

Vitamin C is essential for the formation of antibodies and for aiding recovery after an infection or illness. It helps to form collagen, which is needed for the body's connective tissue. It is also needed for the absorption of iron and for producing haemoglobin and adrenaline. Lack of vitamin C leads to bleeding gums, poor teeth, low resistance to disease and slow recovery from illness.

VITAMIN D (CALCIFEROL)

Vitamin D helps the body to absorb and regulate its intake of calcium and phosphorus, and is needed for strong

bones, teeth and gums. It is absorbed through sunlight as
well as food. Lack of vitamin D causes softening of the
bones and, in severe cases, rickets.

VITAMIN E (TOCOPHEROL)
Vitamin E protects vitamin A and the unsaturated fats in the
body from harmful oxidation. It also assists in healing after
injury or illness. Lack of vitamin E causes muscular wasting,
abnormal fat deposits and abnormal red blood cells.

VITAMIN K (PHYTOMENADIONE)
Vitamin K is essential for blood clotting. Lack of vitamin
K can lead to internal and external bleeding.

EIGHT ESSENTIAL ELEMENTS
Of the nutrients listed above, there are seven elements
essential for life. These are vitamins A, B, C and D, iodine,
sulphur and iron. Citric acid is another element essential
for life. It is a constituent of the metabolic pathway of
the Kreb cycle, which produces energy in the body.
(The Kreb cycle is a very important part of the digestive
system.) Never has there been so much demand for these
substances as supplements, because never before in human
history has our food been cultivated with such artificial
and damaging methods.

CHAPTER FOUR

Foods that Harm, Foods that Heal

I f you suffer from a particular complaint or imbalance —
for example, if you are deficient in a particular mineral,
or if you have difficulty digesting certain kinds of food
— you will need to be given herbal or mineral
supplements by your nutritional therapist. But there are
basic guidelines for healthy eating that apply to all of us.
Once you have become aware of what foods harm and
what foods heal, and revised your eating patterns
accordingly, you will have taken a major step towards
increased well-being.

FOODS THAT HARM

Foods that are detrimental to health, and specifically to the
healthy functioning of the thyroid gland, include refined
white flour, white sugar, heavy salty foods such as crisps
and fries, foods with a high salt content, processed meats
such as frankfurters and meat rolls, and caffeine-rich foods
such as tea, coffee and chocolate.

DISTINGUISHING BETWEEN NATURAL AND REFINED SUGAR

The word sugar has two meanings. Sugar as we have
known it since the middle of the nineteenth century refers
to white sugar, extracted from beet, and brown sugar,
extracted from molasses. If we rely too heavily on refined
foods which contain these sugars, we bypass the needs of
our digestive system, which is designed to work efficiently
to break down whole foods, extracting the goodness from
them for our bodies.

When sugar is consumed in its refined form (as in sweets, drinks, cakes and other processed foods made with white or brown sugar) it does not nourish us — it robs us. Our stores of B vitamins and our all-important bone-building minerals start to leak out from their storage sites. Binge eating can also develop, as the sugar leaves a 'hunger gap', caused by the lack of nutrients.

We may also become addicted to sugar. If eating one small piece of chocolate, cake or biscuit does not satisfy, but leads instead to an endless craving, this indicates the strong possibility of addiction. To break the cycle, it is better gradually to reduce your intake of refined sugar than to cut it out of your diet completely. At the same time, start to introduce foods containing natural sugar into your diet (see below).

PROBLEMS ASSOCIATED WITH EXCESSIVE SUGAR INTAKE

The first victims of excessive sugar intake are our teeth, which suffer from loss of calcium, attack from bacteria and dental caries. Other problems associated with too much refined sugar include: low blood sugar or diabetes; cardiac, arterial and cholesterol problems; acid indigestion; cataracts; hyperactivity; concentration problems; and yeast overgrowth, resulting in candida albicans and other forms of fungal infection, such as vaginal thrush.

NATURAL FORMS OF SUGAR

Simple carbohydrates include sugars which occur as a natural part of food such as milk (lactose), fruit (fructose), grain (maltose), and glucose (found in the blood as a result of digestion). Glucose is the only source of energy that can be used by the brain. A low level of glucose in the blood will cut off supplies to the brain, resulting in feelings of anxiety and faintness, such as in low blood sugar syndrome.

When a good nourishing meal is eaten and digested, there is plenty of glucose available to the brain and the body for energy. Any surplus is converted and stored away in the liver. The store lasts for twenty-four to forty-eight hours. Thereafter, further glucose must be produced from the stores of fat in the body. This source of glucose comes in a 'package'. All the nutrients necessary for digestion and absorption are contained in the milk, the fruit or the grain. Therefore the body is not robbed. These are nutritionally superior foods, which nourish every cell in the body with protein, vitamins, carbohydrates, minerals and fats. (See the Body Eating Clock on page 81.)

Dr Weston Price, a dentist who travelled extensively amongst the peoples of the world who lived on traditional diets, made some wonderful discoveries. His book *Nutrition and Physical Degeneration* shows the before and after effects of modernisation. A simple life, lived in accordance with the natural seasons of the year, eating foods which grow within a certain radius, bestowed good health on the local community. Because of lack of transport, there was no sugar, white flour or tinned food available. There was very little tooth decay. People were vital and healthy. As soon as processed foods became available, problems appeared. There was tooth decay, tuberculosis and difficulty in child bearing. The children were born with poor development of the jaw and the facial structure changed.

OUR BONES, OUR BRAINS, OUR BEHAVIOUR

Protein builds our muscles, our bones and connective tissue. It is involved in the production of hormones such as insulin, digestive enzymes and the formation of antibodies in our immune system. Amino acids (the building blocks of protein, which the body can break down into the various parts) may be involved in the formation of chemicals vital for the brain functions which govern mood and behaviour.

Proteins are one of the absolutely essential ingredients for living a healthy vital life. There is a minimum quantity that we need to eat in order to remain healthy. This quantity depends on our growth rate, body size and the presence or absence of disease.

Our need for protein increases in infancy, during pregnancy and breast-feeding, in healing of the tissues following an accident, injury or operation or when recovering from loss of weight. Our needs for first-class protein increase at a 'crisis' time; in general, we can recover very well with fish, white meat and a little red meat. Traditions of eating across the world have always included such dishes as rice and beans, with added vegetables, herbs and spices, or lentils and barley as in soup, or couscous and chickpeas, whole grain brown bread and baked beans.

THE NEW FOUR FOOD GROUPS

Based on research in America, Japan, Germany, France, England and Ireland, foods are now grouped as follows.

1 *Whole grains* Including whole grain bread, whole grain pasta (made from rice, millet and buckwheat), oats, barley, corn, millet, bulgar wheat, cereal grains, buckwheat, quinoa, spelt grain (the original wheat grain). These grains are rich in fibre, contain some protein, B vitamins and zinc.

2 *Vegetables, fruits and sea vegetables* Excellent sources of body-cleansing fibre, beta carotene and antioxidants to protect the cells in the body from the ravaging effects of pollution, poor diet, stress and tension;

vitamin C and other vitamins and minerals for
whole-body health.

3 *Yoghurt, cheese, cow's milk, sheep, goat or plant milk
   (soya milk, oat milk, rice milk, almond milk or nut milk)*
   Sources of essential fats and fat-soluble vitamins,
   some B vitamins and calcium, magnesium and
   phosphorus.

4 *Beans, peas, lentils, meat, fish, poultry, eggs* Excellent
   sources of fibre from the legumes, also iron, B
   vitamins and minerals. The red meat is distinguished
   as the only source of valuable, easy to obtain
   vitamin B12, which prevents pernicious anaemia.
   Vitamin B12 is essential for nerve health. It
   maintains the integrity of the myelin sheath of the
   spinal cord. Deficiency can cause symptoms such as
   mood disorders, mental slowness, memory defects.
   Smoking (because of the cyanide in tobacco smoke)
   may be implicated in eye problems, because the
   absorption of B12 is interfered with. According to
   research, this happens more in men who smoke
   than in women who do so.

Vegetarians are prime candidates for vitamin B12
deficiency, because their diet is devoid of the most valuable
sources — liver, kidney, muscle meat and some fish. Sea
vegetables or plant sources have to be relied upon for this
vitamin as part of a vegetarian diet. Fish sources are
flounder, herring, mackerel and sardines. Supplementing
the diet with a tonic which contains vitamin B12 is one of
the best ways to guard against this deficiency.

TRADITIONAL DIETS

In the late nineteenth century, Dr Price studied the diet of
the Scottish people. Native people of the Outer Hebrides

ate oaten cakes, fish, eggs, oat porridge, some milk and butter. The Danish, Swiss and southern European people generally lived on black bread, fresh vegetables, fruit, meat infrequently and raw milk. The Peruvian people ate corn beans, seeds, guinea pig meat, seafood, river plants and potatoes.

The early Greeks lived on porridge made of barley meal, lentils, flaxseed, bread, greens, turnips and goat's cheese. Meat was used at celebrations or in war-time only. Hippocrates lived to eighty-three years of age. He understood the needs of the human body instinctively and also through study. Today, we have scientific evidence pouring in to confirm his teachings.

Traditional diets across the world have the following in common:

- the diet is frugal
- the foods are whole food
- the foods are grown locally
- seasonal factors are observed — some foods are scarce at certain times of the year
- no chemicals are used
- cooking methods are slow.

Such diets can be described as being low in calories, protein and fat, and high in complex carbohydrates.

COMPLEX CARBOHYDRATES

Complex carbohydrates are found in grains, beans, seeds, nuts, vegetables and fruits. They are a perfect whole food, containing carbohydrate with some protein, fat, fibre, vitamins, minerals. The grain is revered in all cultures — it is associated with the rise of civilisation all over the world. It comes closer than any other food from

the vegetable kingdom to providing our bodies with all
the building blocks, energy and fibre we need for our
health. After the introduction of oats, rice, millet or
corn to the diet, it takes only a few weeks for the
complex carbohydrates to begin to exhibit their
wonderful properties.

THE BENEFITS OF COMPLEX CARBOHYDRATES

The fibrous part of grains, beans, seeds, nuts, vegetables
and fruits cause a change in the stools — in the west,
stools tend to be small, hard and infrequent. This may be
implicated in diverticular disease, irritable bowel syndrome
or constipation, which afflicts so many people today.
A diet combining whole grain beans, peas, seeds, nuts,
vegetables and fruit produces a profound change in the
colon and texture of the stool. A large, soft, easily
propelled stool is the result.

The bran part of the complex carbohydrate (rice
bran, oat bran, wheat bran, soya bran) has been
recommended by many doctors for helping to maintain
a healthy cholesterol, thereby reducing levels of strokes
and heart problems. Because fibre is so low in calories
and high in bulk, it produces a full feeling and prevents
over-eating. In addition, as the foodstuffs mentioned
here provide the body with the B-complex vitamins
and minerals, they support it in times of stress. They
also provide the body with stamina, both mental and
physical, because of the gentle, steady, slow release of
sugar (glucose).

These foods need to be chewed very well, in order to
release the enzymes in the mouth which prepare them for
easy digestion all the way through the digestive tract. As they
are chewed, they become sweet, satisfying and comforting.

FAT IS ESSENTIAL FOR LIFE

The body needs fat, but it also needs to receive fat in its
most nutritious form. Saturated fat, which is contained
in meat and dairy products, can cause high cholesterol;
unsaturated fats need to be included in the diet as well.
Unsaturated fats come in two forms. Most obviously,
they are present in oils — for example, olive oil, sunflower
oil, soya oil, butter, lard and cocoa butter. They are also
an integral part of certain foods, especially whole grains,
nuts, seeds and fish.

We depend upon fat to deliver the fat-soluble
vitamins A, D, E and K throughout the body. They carry
out protective functions, which prevent infections, skin
lesions, poor circulation, night blindness and 'dry eye'.
They are instrumental in the formation of strong teeth
and healthy gums resistant to gum disease, and in the
production and maintenance of healthy mucous
membrane. All of them are helpful, along with the
B-complex vitamins, for normal growth and development
in babies, young children and teenagers. These vitamins
are like busy mothers and fathers in the body — building,
helping growth, protecting, forming new healthy cells,
preventing severe bleeding and nourishing the cells.

THE FRIENDLY ESSENTIAL FATS

We need to recall the most important functions of fat in
our food: it is a builder. Every cell in our body and brain
has fat as the major component of the cell wall. The fats
called essential fats give our cells impermeable walls,
which we need to keep out the viruses which surround us.
By having regular meals composed of grains, vegetables
and fish, we supply our cells with these vital substances.
Medical science is discovering that these essential fats are

an integral part of unprocessed, naturally grown, chemical-free foods.

THE HEALING FATS

They have different functions in the body. The evening primrose plant, the beautiful borage herb and blackcurrants all provide GLA (gamma linoleic acid). Amongst the many functions it performs are improved circulation, reduction of inflammation and lowering of blood pressure in the arteries. It prevents cholesterol production, helps the T-lymphocytes in the immune system and enables us to burn fat instead of storing it.

Fish is a better source of these fats than meat. Evening primrose oil is recommended by doctors for skin problems, including dry skin, dandruff, dermatitis and eczema. Doctors acknowledge that the faulty metabolism of essential fats, or a deficiency due to a poor diet, is at the root of many of the problems they see daily in their practices. Many of the people who have suffered from psychiatric, behavioural, learning and menstrual problems, in addition to recurring viral or bacterial infections, have been restored to normal life by a prescription of the essential fatty acids both in the diet and in the form of evening primrose, borage or blackcurrant seed oils.

HOW FAT SUPPORTS LIFE

Apart from the medicinal aspects of fat in our diet, fat has other roles to play. Fat adds warmth, comfort and taste to our cooking. It keeps us warm by raising our temperature in cold weather. Our body contours are provided by fat. It also acts as a vital reserve should our food supplies fail. Of the eight essential elements, our vitamin A and E come from the fat in our diet. When we eat a whole food diet, including a wide range of foods, these vitamins, the ordinary fats and the essential fats are all present.

HOW TO ACHIEVE BALANCE

Replace refined sugar with fruit, including: dried fruit; honey; maple syrup; raw cane sugar for cooking (in very reduced amounts); fruit purées and juices and carrot juice for baking. Replace heavy, fatty foods with grilled, low-fat foods, and replace red meat with vegetarian sausages and burgers. Introduce whole grain rice, millet, couscous or bulgar wheat instead of chips. Chips are to be regarded as an occasional treat. Instead of buying ready-made soups and sauces, make your own.

The ideal diet contains approximately twenty-five per cent fat, fifteen per cent protein and sixty per cent carbohydrates. As you adjust your eating habits to obtain this balance, the new foods and extra water will act like brooms and brushes. Waste products which have been clogging up the cells for years will begin to move out through the normal channels of excretion, mainly the kidneys and the intestines. You may experience a feeling of being starving, and not being able to wait for your next meal. This is because the body simply cannot get enough of the delicious, nutritious food. This hunger does not last too long, though, as you begin to efficiently digest, absorb and fuel the body from it in a few weeks. This is the food the brain and body need — they love it!

About one quarter of our diet needs to contain fat. If we consider the foods which are natural bearers of healthy fats, then we are on our way. Sunflower, sesame and pumpkin seeds are excellent sources; when shopping for oil, buy sunflower oil — look for unrefined, cold-pressed varieties, in dark containers. Buy only small quantities and use very little in cooking. Use mainly as dressing on salads.

As your body adjusts to less fat, it also learns to utilise new sources of proteins — less from processed foods, more from fish, home-cooked vegetable and meat soups and stir-fry foods. It is adapting to a greater variety of grains, brown rice, millet, corn (which supply some protein, a little fat and plenty of carbohydrate). The protein we eat becomes the building blocks of the brain and body.

HEALTH-GIVING FATS

The avocado has lots of fibre and is a wonderful source of vitamins, A, C, E and B complex, in addition to minerals and potassium. Avocados help as part of a healthy diet to keep our circulation and heart supplied with excellent nutrition. Very good for the skin, they help to make collagen (which is under our skin), and help to maintain the elasticity and smooth, wrinkle-free appearance of our largest body organ.

Oily fish such as sardines, mackerel and herring are renowned as 'brain food', helping brain function, eyesight and learning ability, reducing cholesterol, thinning the blood and reducing the risk of blood clotting. Fish also helps to balance the body's water levels.

Nuts such as almonds, hazelnuts, chestnuts, walnuts and Brazil nuts contain fats with life-giving enzymes, selenium, B complex, potassium, zinc, calcium, folic acid and iron. Only buy them from a source which has rapid turnover; otherwise, buy them in their shells.

VITAMINS WHICH FEED THE BRAIN

Our brain is the great broadcasting station upon which we depend. All our learning abilities, our creativity, our five senses, are the daily transmissions of this great organ. How do we keep ourselves orientated towards a positive, healthy brain with a good memory, good concentration and retention, socially outgoing, feeling warm and caring towards our family and friends? The answer is simple — feed the brain.

Much has been said about the needs of the body. When we nourish the body with mineral — and vitamin-rich nutrition, certain organs, such as the liver, and the muscles become depots for the storage of energy. This is a miracle of economy by the body. The stored energy (called glycogen) can be called upon to help in a situation the body sees as an emergency — too long between meals, an injury, accident or emotional upheaval. However, should we, through lack of awareness and conscious thought about the needs of our body, cause this to occur frequently we will notice the effects: easily fatigued or easily injured muscles, muscle cramp and restless legs are just some of the problems of depletion of nutrition in the muscular body.

The brain has no such storage depots — it has no capacity to store energy. It needs to receive a constant supply of fuel from the blood. The heart pumps one quarter of its blood directly to the brain. If your meal has been poorly chosen — composed of white sugar, high fat, high salt, low in fibre, complex carbohydrates and essential fatty acids — the blood carries this nutrient-poor supply to the brain. This may be sufficient to deplete the brain of the constant supply of nourishing minerals, vitamins, enzymes, amino acids, glucose and oxygen necessary for it to do its work.

FOODS THAT FEED THE BRAIN

Phosphorus-rich foods include the most well-known source — fish, also a rich source of iron, iodine, sulphur and zinc. Other important sources of phosphorus are almonds, protein drink made from soya flour (available in health shops), beans, cheese, wheat germ, wheat bran (from organically grown sources, so that the bran does not have to compete for nutrients with pesticides), sunflower seeds, cashew nuts, Brazil nuts, whole soya beans (from an organically grown source only, to avoid genetically engineered foods).

WINTER FOODS RICH IN IMMUNE-PROTECTING VITAMINS AND MINERALS

Vitamin A (beta carotene) Yellow, deep orange and dark green vegetables and fruit.

Vitamin B complex Almonds, whole grains, meat, poultry, cheese, fish, sunflower seeds, eggs, avocado, rice bran.

Vitamin B12 Beef, beef liver (from free-range sources), eggs, flounder, herring, mackerel, milk, milk products, sardines.

Vitamin B9 (folic acid) Barley, calf's liver (free-range), beans, chickpeas, green leaf vegetables, lentils, whole grain rice, peas, split peas, sprouted seeds, wheat, wheat germ.

Vitamin C Acerola cherries, blackcurrants, fruit, rosehip, broccoli, cabbage, parsley, potatoes, tomatoes, paprika, sprouts, lemons, watercress.

Vitamin D Cod liver oil, salmon, sardines, tuna, butter, milk, eggs, cheese.

Vitamin E All unprocessed seeds and nuts, whole unprocessed grains, green vegetables, evening primrose oil, borage oil, cold-pressed oils used as dressings in salads — soya bean, safflower, wheat germ.

Bioflavonoids Skin and pulp of fruits such as oranges, lemons, apricots and cherries, buckwheat, green pepper.

Calcium Sesame seeds, tahini, hummus, fish, yoghurt, cheese, milk, sea vegetables (carrageen, dulse, kombu, wakame), black strap molasses, kelp, tofu, leafy green vegetables, almonds, sunflower seeds.

Iron Meat, egg yolk, sea vegetables, black strap molasses, chickpeas, lentils, mussels, pistachios, pumpkin seeds, walnuts, wheat germ.

Magnesium Almonds, fish, leafy green vegetables, black strap molasses, nuts and seeds, soya beans, wheat germ (many foods that are rich in calcium also have magnesium).

Phosphorus Skimmed milk, wheat germ, soya flour, brown rice, wholemeal bread, almonds, dried beans, free-range calf's liver, cheese, eggs, fish, peas, poultry, seeds, sardines, tuna, whole grains.

Silica Oats, soya beans, sesame, sunflower and pumpkin seeds, black strap molasses.

Zinc All unprocessed whole grains, meat, poultry, fish, egg yolk, turkey, oysters, wheat germ, oat bran.

CHAPTER FIVE

Consulting a Nutritional Therapist

DO I NEED NUTRITIONAL THERAPY?

How do you know whether you would benefit from nutritional therapy? The short answer is that everyone, whatever their state of health, is likely to benefit to some extent from looking carefully at their eating habits and improving them as necessary. If you suddenly experience a change of health for the worse, such as the development of asthma, migraine or insomnia, these are clear messages from your body that you need to reconsider both your eating habits and your lifestyle. On the other hand, many illnesses do not present themselves suddenly.

These are some indicators that your health is being undermined:

1 *Fatigue* This form of tiredness is not alleviated by rest. Even when you go to bed early and appear to sleep well, you wake up feeling tired.

2 *Irritability* We are all irritable on occasions, but this is different. If you are chronically irritable, it means you become irritable for very little or no reason at all, probably due to a hormonal imbalance.

3 *Change of appetite* Eating too little or eating too much can lead to great weight loss or gain.

4 *Energy loss* If your energy is low, your immune system will be vulnerable, lowering your resistance to infection. You will be susceptible to regular colds and flu, especially in winter.

5 *Collapse* Following a heart attack or irritable bowel syndrome, arthritis, diabetes, asthma or other illness which necessitates a visit to hospital.

If any of these states describes you, it is advisable for you to seek the help of a professional nutritionist.

FINDING A NUTRITIONAL THERAPIST

Once you have decided to consult a nutritional therapist, how do you set about finding one? The best way is probably by recommendation; seek advice from your local health store or library if you do not have friends who can put you in touch with someone they recommend. Failing that, consult your local directory or contact one of the organisations listed in Helpful Addresses.

WILL VISITING A NUTRITIONIST AFFECT ANY MEDICATION I AM TAKING?

No. But if you are taking any medication, it is important that you give this information to your nutritionist. It will also help your nutritionist if you have recently had a full medical diagnosis, as this can narrow down the time it takes to identify the source of your problem. Nutritional therapy can work extremely effectively alongside orthodox medicine. If you have a medical check up before visiting a nutritionist, you will probably find it interesting to have a follow-up one a few months later, so that you and your doctor can establish the effects of your nutritionist's treatment.

WHAT HAPPENS IN THE INITIAL SESSION?

When you meet your nutritional therapist for the first time, the consultation will probably last for an hour to an hour and a half. To gain a better understanding of your present needs, the therapist is likely to ask quite detailed questions about your personal history. You may be asked to describe your past as well as current lifestyle, including your eating patterns and your attitude towards yourself.

You may also be asked about your family's health history. This is because we all carry genetic weaknesses as well as strengths. It is true that within the same family each person is completely unique, with specific needs. At the same time, however, we all inherit tendencies which we may be able to reverse once we become fully aware of them. Looking at your family history may show that you have inherited problems such as being overweight, skin problems, constipation, poor circulation, chilblains or feeling the cold even in warm weather. Just because your ancestors suffered from these complaints does not mean you have to carry them with you through your own life.

THE THREE CATEGORIES OF ASSESSMENT

The three categories of assessment that I observe as a nutritional therapist are as follows.

1 *A thorough physical assessment* Includes: a physical appraisal, noting any current weaknesses or symptoms, such as backache, headache, indigestion, breathing difficulties, etc., as well as a note of what form of exercise you take on a regular basis.

2 *An assessment of your family's health history* This includes siblings, parents and grandparents; your personal health history from birth to the present, including recurrent patterns of illness or repeating symptoms, record of drugs, medication or vitamins used, including the periods of time over which they have been used.

3 *Dietary information* Record what you ate as a young person growing up, which will give an indication of your ancestors' way of eating, as well as what you typically eat now.

4 *Blood, urine or hair analysis* Your therapist may take samples and explain the results of the laboratory analysis at your next appointment.

CREATING AN EATING REGIME

Together, you and your nutritionist will work out a revised eating regime, which may include mineral or vitamin supplements, depending on your state of health and lifestyle, and also the nature of your specific problem. To do this, you will be asked to consider food in the widest sense, and to write out a brief account of what you are likely to eat over a period of a week. It is important that you do this as accurately as possible, because your account will reveal any strengths and weaknesses you may have both in the choices you make and in the way and the time you usually eat.

If your nutritionist suspects an allergy, you may wait until your second appointment to establish the results of a blood, urine or hair analysis, which will have identified the particular allergy. Depending on the extent to which your current eating habits are conducive to health, and on your condition, the changes in your diet may be significant and immediate or gradual. This is something that you and your nutritionist are likely to work on together, but a typical change of shopping list will look like the following.

Old Shopping List	**New Shopping List**
White bread	Wholemeal or granary bread
Cereal	Sugar-free muesli
French loaves	Mixed seed loaves
Brown bread	Caraway seed rye bread
Black tea	Low-caffeine or herbal tea
Instant coffee	Fresh coffee

Old Shopping List	New Shopping List
White sugar	Barbados sugar
Buns and cakes	Whole grain biscuits
Biscuits	Nuts and dried fruit
Chocolate	Carob
Meat	White fish
Fish in batter	Oil-rich fish (salmon, mackerel)
Chicken	Free-range chicken
Butter	Cold-pressed virgin oils
Whole-fat milk	Skimmed milk
Canned vegetables	Fresh, organic vegetables
Fruit	Fruit in season only
Jam	Sugar-free fruit spreads
Ready-made desserts	Live yoghurt

THE IMPORTANCE OF EATING REGULARLY

One of the keys to good nutrition is eating regularly and having balanced meals. Your nutritionist will probably encourage you to eat a good breakfast, a lunch which contains plenty of fresh vegetables and a light supper. If your caffeine intake is high, you will be advised to cut down on it and in some cases to eliminate it. If you drink a lot of alcohol, you will be asked to reduce your intake.

Many simple problems, such as mood swings and low energy levels, are caused by a diet which is high in refined sugar and does not include a sufficient range of protein-rich foods. If this is the case with you, you will probably be advised to include protein-rich drinks or snacks in your daily eating programme, as well as a good breakfast, lunch and evening meal. Every person's eating requirements are unique, but for a typical, nutritious daily menu, see page 105.

EXERCISE

If exercise is not part of your current lifestyle, your
nutritionist will almost certainly recommend at least a
twenty-minute walk each day. Regular exercise improves
the metabolism and increases mental alertness. If you
exercise well, you will start to digest your food more
efficiently and to sleep more deeply. Health, like illness,
does not affect particular organs in isolation — it affects
the whole person. Regular exercise plays an important
part in maintaining a healthy lifestyle.

AFFIRMATIONS

As you revise your eating habits and your attitude to life,
you may find it helpful to use affirmations to confirm
yourself in your work. Affirmations are a simple, yet
effective, way of bringing about a long-term change of
attitude and in helping to banish old habits. They should
focus on your present state; affirmations are not wishes!
  I find them most effective if they are repeated daily, on
waking each morning and just before going to sleep in
the evening. Typical affirmations about health are:
      'I am expressing myself in positive ways.'
      'I feel light and buoyant and full of hope.'
      'I am becoming stronger and healthier every day.'

HOW MANY SESSIONS WILL I NEED?

The amount of sessions will depend on the nature of
your problem, and on your ability to change your
lifestyle in order to relieve the problem. It is impossible
to say in advance how many sessions a person will need,
because everyone is unique. Even if two people with
similar lifestyles and family histories came to me with
the same problem, I would not assume that they would

both need the same treatment over the same period
of time.

As the weeks progress, you will find that a great
deal of nutritional therapy turns on your ability to help
yourself. Your nutritionist is there to advise and guide you,
but in the end you will be the one to ring the changes.

CHAPTER SIX

Monitoring Progress

C hanging old, ingrained eating habits can be a challenging experience. To help keep up your morale, and to monitor your progress as accurately as possible, it is recommended that you keep a daily food diary over a period of at least three months. Some changes in diet will have an immediate effect. As the effects of certain foods are cumulative, however, benefits from these will occur at a deep level only with time. The changes your nutritionist recommends should not be seen as a short-term fix, but as the start of a change in your relationship to food that should last for life. So bear in mind both the long-term and the short-term value of the food you are eating when you start your diary.

KEEPING A FOOD DIARY

Use your food diary to record:

- what you eat and drink, including quantity
- how you eat (with enthusiasm, resistance, enjoyment, quickly or slowly)
- the effects of what you eat — immediately after the meal and a few hours later.

As well as keeping this record, it can help to assess your overall attitude to food after the first couple of weeks. Your self-assessment may look something like this.

LIFESTYLE AND FOOD

Old Thoughts	New Thoughts
Food was a means to an end, given little or no thought, as long as I had	A new awareness of the importance of food in my motto 'I need quality not

Old Thoughts	**New Thoughts**
enough energy to get through my day	quantity'; I want fresh food, which has higher amounts of the vitamins, minerals and enzymes needed to keep me healthy
Food was chosen for convenience, speed of preparation, minimum time spent at the cooker	I take pleasure in cooking with care and adding herbs to my meals
No association made between outbreaks of flu, colds, infections and the food being consumed	When I feel a cold coming on, I eat lots of fresh fruit and it goes away
Liquid intake meant copious cups of tea, occasional coffee or alcohol, fruit juices, high-caffeine drinks	Liquid intake means a glass of water at least three times a day; my new foods provide a lot of liquid also
Favourite foods were on my shopping list every day, including ones which were high in fat, sugar, salt, flavourings, additives, colourings, preservatives and, unknown to me, herbicides, pesticides, antibiotics, hormones and irradiation	I now look for 'no artificial anything' on food labels — including sweeteners, sugar, salt, flavours, colour or preservatives

Practising Self-Observation

Look out for signs of deficiency in your diet. Do you look pale? Do you feel tired? Do you feel breathless after climbing up the stairs? If so, you need more folic acid, iron and foods rich in B12. These include all kinds of greens, and a little meat.

Because you are in a transitional phase in the first few months, your body is feeling the changes. Gradually, you will build up sufficient minerals, vitamins and essential fatty acids. These will strengthen not only your immune system but the trillions of cells that make you who you are — you will develop much greater resistance to colds and flu.

Honouring the Digestive Process

Even a nutritionally rich meal can be undermined if it is not eaten in the right spirit. The following guidelines are basic to good digestion, and were once widely practised:

1 *Quietness before starting to eat* This was achieved in the past by having a quiet drink and a prayer before meals.

2 *Eating with enjoyment, awareness and gratitude* In households where people love food, great discussion on the subject takes place.

3 *A half-hour period of rest or quiet after the meal* Rushing back to work, brisk walking, heavy labouring work, playing any game in which there is strenuous physical activity and/or which involves keen concentration, all interfere with the proper digestion and assimilation of food.

Relaying Progress to your Nutritionist

Bring your food diary and any related notes to your appointments. Your nutritionist may be able to make

connections that are not immediately apparent to you. He
or she will also look at your overall health picture. Are you
feeling less tired? Have you better, more steady energy during
the day? Are your moods better? All of these questions are
as important whether you are a man, woman or child.

Your diary will be of enormous help in reminding
you how you were feeling six weeks ago compared with
how you are now. Are you sleeping better, waking up
refreshed? Although it may take three months to achieve
correct balance throughout the hormonal system, good
signs — such as less cravings for sugar, caffeine or nicotine,
less bloating, less fluid retention — should become
apparent after the first four to six weeks. Your body
temperature should be stable and your circulation good.
Your hair, nails and teeth should become stronger.

ADJUSTING TO YOUR NEW EATING PROGRAMME

Most people take quite a long time to feel comfortable with
a new way of eating. After about six weeks, however, you
should begin to feel quite relaxed with your programme.
You have now become expert at label reading; shopping has
a new function: to protect you from choosing incorrectly or
unwisely. Recipes should be simply prepared, cooked
according to your time available, and served quickly to
enjoy all the benefits. You may be missing your sweet treats.
You may need either to make your own or to try the
delicatessen and health shops for home-made, rich-in-fibre,
low-sugar muffins, carrot cake, etc. Look for the yoghurts
containing lactobacillus bulgarius.

THE SWISS NATURE DOCTOR

Dr Vogel, the famous Swiss nature doctor, was born in
1902 and has been a practitioner since the 1930s. He

has been responsible for much of the now widespread knowledge available on the subject of eating the 'whole food way'. His book *The Nature Doctor* has sold 2,000,000 copies, and has been published in many languages; it is the story of Vogel's life, detailing how he discovered the medicinal power of herbs, descriptions of how they work in the body and his herbal tincture formulations.

One of Dr Vogel's many discoveries was made while working with clients in his clinic in Teufen in Appenzellerland. There he prepares extracts from fresh plants and uses them as medicine. He found that the tinctures made from the juice rather than the dried plant were more effective. Your nutritionist will choose from a wide variety of such herbal plants to help you. In the early stages of your eating-for-health programme, it will be necessary to use these herbs, and perhaps mineral and vitamin supplements, to encourage the immune system to become strong.

Sample Food Diary
Day One, Week One

Old Breakfast	New Breakfast
Refined cereal (low in fibre), white bread, marmalade, tea or coffee.	Cereal (high in fibre, low in sugar), rice cakes with sunflower spread, sugar-free apricot jam, low-tannin, low-caffeine tea or coffee.
11.00 am	**11.00 am**
Craving for something sweet or salty, also longing for tea or coffee.	Have protein drink — feel quite nourished, have more energy, better concentration, better mood.

Day One, Week One *contd.*

1.30 pm Lunch

Shop-bought sandwich — cheese, egg mayonnaise (high in fat) and a tinned fizzy drink (high in sugar).

1.30 pm Lunch

The protein drink's effects have lasted until now. This means I have got through the morning since breakfast with the minimum discomfort and the minimum of snacks and high-caffeine drinks. My healthier morning has helped me to choose a healthier lunch, to eat slowly, to enjoy and appreciate my meal. It was easier to choose yoghurt instead of a rich dessert with creams. I enjoy meat, vegetables, gravy for lunch and choose a yoghurt for dessert.

4.00 pm

Feeling peckish. Would love a bar of chocolate.

4.00 pm

Have protein drink, and have a high-fibre, high-protein bar to help me steer clear of the chocolate.

5.00 pm

On the way home from work — tired, peckish.

5.00 pm

Have bottled water in the car. Eat protein bar — feel better.

Day One, Week One *contd.*

6.30 pm Dinner

Usually something fast, such as pizza or Chinese take-away or fish and chips. Fresh vegetables are reserved for weekends, when there is time to cook. Will make an effort to have a small amount of salad.

6.30 pm Dinner

Brought home quiche lorraine from the delicatessen, with two salads — broccoli with cashew nuts and pasta with celery, cucumber, peas and corn. After dinner I allow myself a packet of crisps as a treat. Feeling good.

END OF WEEK ONE

I have had a reasonably good week. Made a good effort to keep to the programme. Found the protein drink a life-saver! Could not have managed the discipline of keeping away from the refined sugars without it. The protein drink not only gave me a nice nourished feeling, but it seems to have reduced the severity of the withdrawal symptoms from sugar in general. I did have to have a bar of chocolate three times during the week, but I went to the local health shop and bought a healthier alternative. I needed the chocolate when I ran out of supplies. Shopping is not easy when you are learning to read labels. A helpful hint — *never* go shopping when you are hungry! Do not bring either yourself or the children to shop until you have taken the edge off your appetite.

Day One, Week Two
Breakfast

I am loving my breakfast. This week I am having fresh fruit in season, with natural yoghurt and a little fruit yoghurt. I add sunflower seeds and hazelnuts for extra nourishment.

Day One, Week Two *contd.*

11.00 am

I make my protein drink up with water and juice. I have my normal lunch, because it is familiar and comforting.

4.00 pm

This is definitely my low-energy time. The protein drink and bar are very helpful.

6.30 pm Dinner

A vegetable dish with breast of chicken is quick and tasty.

END OF WEEK FIVE

Have become quite an expert at label reading, so my 'new' shopping is a lot easier. I have found some new substitute foods for old ones. There is a very good selection, for example, of muesli–type breakfast cereals. I have chosen a very basic one and add my own fresh fruit to it, with pumpkin seeds. There are many types of bread, including granary grain bread, oat bread, rye bread and whole grain crispbreads with sesame seeds. Sometimes I have feta cheese, cottage cheese or vegetarian cheese instead of butter. My whole interest in food is changing — I am looking out for a much wider range than ever before. Consequently, my approach to my programme has changed. This is an education in eating, not at all the narrow diet that I thought would be my prescription.

Day One, Week Six

Breakfast

A glass of warm water. My nutritional counsellor has now recommended this as a great way to start the day. Muesli, fruit, pumpkin seeds, granary bread, vegetarian cheese.

11.00 am

Protein drink, crackers with sesame seeds (just in case!).

Day One, Week Six *contd.*

1.30 pm Lunch

I now choose extra vegetables to have with fish, chicken or meat. Most days a yoghurt, occasionally fruit salad with cream.

4.00 pm

Protein drink. I keep my high-protein bar for the journey home, because it stops me going into the shop for a bar of chocolate. I also have a handful of sunflower seeds.

6.30 pm Dinner

Lasagne with salad and wholemeal pasta.

THE IMPORTANCE OF KEEPING A FOOD DIARY

Keeping a diary will enhance your sense of responsibility towards yourself; the combined knowledge of choosing healthier food and changing your eating habits will give you a feeling of being in control of your life. Gradually the cravings will disappear. You will start to appreciate your lunch and dinner more if they are thoughtfully prepared, well-balanced dishes rather than fast food.

RECOMMENDED FOODS

Chickpeas; home-made brown bread with added rice bran, oat bran or wheat germ; flapjacks with added molasses (made from oat flakes, honey, sunflower oil, molasses with sunflower seeds and sesame seeds added); pumpkin seeds; almonds; parsley; cress; sprouted alfalfa seeds; sprouted mung beans — small but very valuable sources of a whole range of vitamins, minerals and iron.

CHAPTER SEVEN

Nutrition and the Environment

When you feel quite well, having reached the stage where you are really enjoying your food, a new development takes place. Questions arise. What is in my food? How can I be assured of the quality of my food? How and where is it grown? You will want less colourings, less preservatives. You will certainly not want food that has been chemically treated, genetically engineered, treated with hormones or irradiated.

Transporting and storing food had been a concern for every society since man stopped hunting and gathering. Both staples and luxury foods have always been processed for journeys beyond the stockade — or the grave. Every army has devised ways of carrying its rations and many of their techniques we still use today.

The Moghuls moved across Asia with flanks of salted meat strapped to their pack animals, and yak's milk in hides became cheese as the animals plodded along. The American plains Indians dried buffalo meat, which they secured in strips for when it was needed; this is still available as 'beef jerky', from when their technique was commercialised. Salted fish was taken on board boats in the days before refrigeration, but it remains in the diet of seafarers, even after they pull up anchor and become landlubbers.

More spectacularly, Napoleon Bonaparte took his cooks to war with him. That way they were on hand to honour his victories with new dishes such as 'chicken Marengo' or 'chicken Kiev'. He knew his soldiers marched on their stomachs, and he employed good psychology.

CHEMICAL FARMING

Chemical farming came into being with a great flourish
around 1945, but was really being developed since 1918.
With the use of mineral fertilisers rich in nitrogen,
phosphorus and potassium, farming became a profitable
business — agribusiness. Until then, agriculture had been
mostly carried out on nature's terms. Man had cooperated
with the earth. The farming was based on the needs of the
soil — the variety and rotation of crops, rest periods, and
feeding the soil with compost or manure. Only a small
number of traditional farmers remain at the end of the
twentieth century. Their focus changed from feeding the
locality to answering the needs of the food conglomerates.

The farmer of one hundred years ago knew by
following the tradition of his forefathers that his methods
were enriching, sustainable and safeguarding the future
of the soil. Today, we have a farmer who produces
technological food — and a confused consumer. It is
time for consumers to ask the question: where does
responsibility for the safety of our food begin?

PROFIT MARGINS

In a quest for even greater profit margins, scientists are
ready to unleash their latest discoveries on the world:
genetically changed plants and vegetables, programmed to
grow and behave exactly the way scientists want them to.

The story of the American breakfast food is that of
the promulgation of the western diet. In the mid–1800s,
a popular quick breakfast food was sold in small navy blue
tubs, with the picture of a smiling Quaker on them; the
connotations were of thrift, piety and colonic hygiene.
Simple and regular. The Kellogg brothers then 'invented'
cornflakes, however; because they were soon in

competition with each other, they had to invent ever more appealing packs.

Psychological appeal features from here on in the packaging and marketing. Eventually, the boxes became huge and brightly coloured, with plastic 'extras' inside and smiling Quakers replaced with *fun*. So our food comes to us now from the silo, wrapped in plastic, and we eat it on the run or whenever we want to enjoy ourselves. The early pioneers of these foods have become corporate America, which in turn is part of world conglomerates. They are now more involved in marketing and political lobbying than nourishing the nation.

Four multinational companies now control eighty-seven per cent of the world tobacco trade; three control eighty-five per cent of the tea trade; three control eighty-three per cent of the cocoa trade; three control eighty per cent of the banana business; and five control seventy-seven per cent of the grain trade. Unlike governments, they are accountable to no one.

According to Paul Ross, in *World* magazine of November 1996,

> Today's unjust food trade system began in colonial times, when export or cash crops were given priority over subsistence crops that fed the local people. Profit margins have become the focus, and it will stay that way even though production is awry. We have mountains of food wasting away, or going to animal fodder, while people hunger everywhere. The old practice of subsidising farmers to stop them producing too much will probably be phased out soon as farmers give up their way of life.

Two new practices are being introduced by the mass producers of food, with only a cynical eye to the profit margin and no thought to the health of the public or the environment. Because of protests about preservatives in food, some producers now protect their crops by irradiating them. This practice is questioned by Dr Mindell:

The purpose is to kill bacteria, fungi, insects and many undesirable creatures that may spread disease. The food does not become radioactive; however, irradiation does cause other changes in the molecular structure of food, notably an increase in free radicals (the unstable molecules that can cause other cells to mutate) and the formation of other potentially carcinogenic chemicals.

The other new threat looming on the horizon is food from genetically engineered crops.

BRINGING IN THE HARVEST

The world's demand for maize was once met by the USA, but now China exports maize at the expense of its soya-bean crop. Meanwhile, in the USA, the maize-poor soil has been planted with soya beans as this is a leguminous plant that restores nitrogen to the ground.

The soya bean, revered in the east for centuries as 'meat with no bones', was the first food to be engineered. In autumn 1996, they brought in the harvest in Missouri. The first genetically engineered crops were not openly identified as such — although they could have been, at source — and once they came into the market place, they could not be distinguished from the normal crop.

Talk Radio, in December 1996, posed the question: do we want this crop on our dinner table? The guest protesting against 'gene-tinkering' was Dr Richard Lacey of Leeds University, and he was supported by many of those who called in to the programme. Dr Lacey's argument was that this crop had not been tested. Surely, he argued, it was possible to do damage to growing organisms by feeding them material that had had its DNA manipulated to react to its normal environment in unpredictable ways. Going against the laws of nature meant nature might *not* heal anymore — where once meat was good, for example, it now meant BSE killed people. What would genetically altered food do to us? We don't know. So let's find out *before* we all eat it unknowingly.

Greenpeace tried to stop the cargo boats, and the World Food summit in India was interrupted by protesters who claimed it could be a catastrophic mistake to allow genetically engineered food into our food chain.

CONSUMER CHOICE

In Europe, 2,000 miles away, it looks as if consumers will not be given the choice. There will be no labelling to indicate the fact that the soya bean is different. They will only be a very tiny percentage of the main crop, which is how they will be incorporated into the food chain. Foods that are expected to come into the market place soon are: maize (insect-protected maize); oil-seed rape (herbicide-tolerant); tomatoes and tomato paste (slow-ripening and non-squashy); sugar beet (herbicide-resistant); and cotton (bollworm-resistant). Others in the pipeline are chicory, tobacco, squash, canola, papaya, flax and brewer's yeast.

Research in Denmark has shown that genetically engineered resistance to a herbicide in oil-seed rape was transferred to weeds, which then passed it on to the next generation. Genetically engineered oil-seed rape is one of three crops which have been approved for Britain, the other two being the soya bean and maize. Already it has emerged that genetic engineering could result in crops that are harmful to health. When the Brazil nut was genetically transferred (i.e. through genetic engineering) to the soya bean, it was quickly found to be allergenic — that is, anyone allergic to nuts was also allergic to the soya bean. This project has since been abandoned.

SILENT SPRING

Silent Spring, a classic study of the effects of pesticides, was published in North America and Britain in the 1960s. Rachel Carson was the first woman to draw to the attention of the unsuspecting public the dangers of DDT. She named twenty-three other herbicides and pesticides as equally destructive to the life cycle of the soil, the creatures which lived on the plants from the soil, their reproductive cycle and the consequences for the new generation. Since then, hundreds more chemicals have been introduced, and now amongst the public there is grave concern about the damage caused by them.

WHAT IS IN MY FOOD?

To answer this question, you need to know what *should* be in the soil. Good soil is crumbly in texture. In every inch of the soil there is a living microcosm by which the soil is both aerated and kept moisture-retentive. Tiny passages are created by the insects and earthworms which inhabit rich earth.

THE TISSUE OF THE SOIL

Fungal elements form a web which surrounds and penetrates the structure of plant roots, facilitating the plant's nourishment from the soil. Special soil organisms preserve the ability of the soil to survive the varying temperatures, rainfall, frost or heat of each season. The soil provides the nutrients for plants, which have water, carbon and nitrogen as their main constituents. The carbon material is the woody or fibrous part that, if not eaten by us or those we eat, goes back into the soil and in some circumstances forms the peat or coal we burn. So we turn it into energy we call heat. If we eat this plant material, we turn it into the energy that is 'being alive'.

The nitrogen is held in the fibrous section, and reacts with the hydrogen and oxygen in our water and air, and with sunlight; it forms the green and leafy part of the plant. This, with the stems and roots, holds the vitamins, minerals and trace elements we need to grow our bodies properly.

When we take a plant out of the soil, we are removing material which we must replace if we want that same soil to keep producing for us. Simply to pump it with nitrate fertilisers is not to replenish it properly. This makes for unbalanced soil. We should put compost and manure back into the soil, and let the micro-organisms and weather do the complex job of breaking down the nitrogen and carbon that is needed. Then we should plan our planting and harvesting around crop rotation.

CROP ROTATION

Crop rotation is the three- — or even better, five- — year planting plan a good farmer has for his fields. The same crop is not grown in successive years on the same plot; a waiting period of three to five years ensures that the soil has been 'fed' and has absorbed the nutrients that were first removed with the harvest. In the in-between years, the farmer grows other crops that take a slightly different nutrient balance from the soil.

For example, a nitrogen-hungry plant like sweet corn (maize) is grown one year, with soya bean grown the next year. The beans, like all legumes, have nodules on their roots that store nitrogen the rest of the plant has drawn in. So when the soya beans are harvested, the root is left in the ground; as it breaks down and decays, it leaves a little more nitrogen behind than other plants would — especially the maize plant.

If the farmer planted squash or marrow-like plants after the soya bean, he would be taking very little nitrogen from the soil, because marrow or squashes — as the name implies — are mostly water. This is a pattern of planting perfected by the Indians of Central America a thousand years ago. They not only fed themselves well without chemical fertilisers, but also invented our most famous breakfast food — the cornflake.

The rotation of crops practised by most farmers before the end of the Second World War conserved the fertility of the soil. Tended with smaller machinery and shallow digging tools, the soil increased in depth and fertility almost indefinitely. The top soil became nutrient-rich, and it resisted the climatic tendency to wear it away.

DAMAGE TO THE STRUCTURE OF THE SOIL

Once the application of fertiliser began, there came a great demand on the soil for increased production. Crop yields increased, soil richness decreased and the tissue containing the micro-organisms has been damaged. Worms and insects are fewer in number, the crumb structure has begun to degenerate. The production of high-yielding crops has resulted in stripping the fertility needed for the next generation.

THE DISAPPEARING TOP SOIL

We have lost at least 250 billion tons of top soil into the oceans. We know that 24.7 million kilos of pesticides (or substances containing the ingredients of pesticides) were used in the UK in 1992. The value was £413 million. In the thirty years since Rachel Carson sounded the warning to wild life and to us, there has been a thirty-fold increase in the use of pesticides. The new products may break down more speedily, but they are equally toxic.

The Pesticide Action Network (PAN) has been campaigning for years for the prohibition of the 'Dirty Dozen', including three chemicals identified by Carson and still in use today. The Pesticide Exposure Group of Sufferers has estimated that 2,500 of its 6,000 members have been damaged by organophosphates (OPs), which were developed from nerve gases. They are used mainly in sheep-dipping. Symptoms of mild OP poisoning are flu symptoms, headaches, fatigue, dizziness; acute poisoning can be fatal. The OPs were to be the main chemical which caused disorder in nature, due to the destructive effect on weeds and bacteria. We are now recognising its destructive effect on humans. The top soil which is now in the oceans has taken with it the nutrients necessary to maintain the life cycle of the soil.

QUALITY CONTROL

How can you be assured of the quality of your food? You may be lucky enough to have access to a retail outlet which displays a great deal of information about your food. Clear signs inform you of the farm from which the meat came, how the animals were fed (on grass or feed), the age at which the animals were slaughtered. Of great concern now to the consumer is the manner in which the animals have been reared, whether they have been humanely handled right through their lives. It is quite obvious that there is a difference between animals that are treated well and those that are just a business investment.

FRUITS, VEGETABLES, HERBS AND SPICES

Similar signs are necessary to state from where vegetables and fruit originate. Choices available to you should be:

- no artificial fertiliser residue
- no toxic chemicals used after harvesting
- no cosmetic wax coating
- no artificial colouring
- no irradiation
- no genetic or transgenic engineering
- herbs and spices as nature intended — *natural*.

HOW TO USE YOUR POWER AS A CONSUMER

Constant dialogue with your producer, supermarket manager or local farmer creates a greater awareness of your needs as a consumer. The more people insist on having organic produce in their local shops, the more likely it is that the trends of intensive chemical farming will be reversed. This will safeguard not only your own health, but that of future generations. The soil will then be fertile for generations to come, the cycle of wild life will have established a flourishing habitat and the birds will have returned. The life of the earth will be secured.

RECYCLING, COMPOSTING — AND WHY

In the hot weather of July 1994, I was visiting a friend in
the Midlands of England. I arrived with a large box of
nectarines which I had bought locally — there was a glut,
and they were very inexpensive. They were not UK–
grown, but an EU product, and they tasted wonderful.
My friend told me her pregnant daughter was having
cravings for this fruit and liked to eat five or six a day.
They both decided that it was all right to do so, as this
was fresh fruit. What could be wrong with that?

On the second evening of my visit, we listened with
horror to the evening news: there was a warning that
adults should not eat more than two of these nectarines
per day, and children one every other day, because it had
been widely noted that many people were having allergic
reactions to them. It was presumed the fruit had been
treated with something toxic. In near panic my friend
phoned her daughter — she could only think of the worst
possible scenario for her unborn grandchild.

Alan Gear wrote in the *Henry Doubleday Research
Association (HDRA) Newsletter* in 1993:

> Although there is a great deal of public unease over
> the use of pesticides, few people have first-hand
> experience of acute poisoning by these chemicals.
> The fear is based on the possible harmful effects of
> accumulating pesticide residues over many years of
> eating conventional food and drinking water
> contaminated with pesticides. Such compounds are
> known to cause cancers and genetic damage at
> high doses in laboratory animals. How can we be
> certain they are safe at current levels?

The World Health Organization estimates that every year 3 million suffer acute, severe pesticide poisoning, of which over 20,000 may die. Much of this human tragedy takes place in developing countries where, worldwide, around 25 million people are thought to be adversely affected by sprays one way or another.

Gear had just returned from Venezuela, and gave a short review of the effects of the downturn in the country's fortunes due to the fall in the oil market. As a result of economic need, farmers were encouraged to concentrate on intensive fruit farming. This necessitated big expenditures in chemical treatments to maximise yields. However, the farmers could no longer tolerate the expense involved — both to their finances and to their health.

But it was what they had to say about pesticides that really caught my attention. One farmer reported that over forty people in his village had been poisoned by eating contaminated food. A speaker from Brazil showed a distressing set of slides of babies born to wives of agricultural workers. All had serious birth defects like extra or deformed limbs, or absence of eyes. Of eighty or so Andean farmers in the audience, none used any protective clothing, or took any precautions when spraying. Pesticides were frequently broken down into unlabelled containers. Instructions, even when they could be read, were rarely followed. Many of the chemicals were banned in the west. Is it surprising that human health suffers?

While I was out of the UK, the *Observer* newspaper ran a story alleging a possible link between the fungicidal benomyl, better known to gardeners as Benlate, and clusters of children in Lincolnshire born without eyes. Apparently in a Californian study, 63.5 per cent of pregnant rats dosed with high levels of benomyl and fed on protein-deficient diets, developed severe ocular anomalies.

The seasonal applications of these poisons are not the only source we have to worry about: we must remember they are recycled with crop residues and build up in the soil. The soil could be thought of as the earth's placenta — primitive people would have a clear idea of this as a part of Mother Earth, but for us 'Mother' as a name for the earth has become a cliché. Yet the earth's soil, water and atmosphere nourish us and recycle our waste so we can feed again. We all know what happens to the embryo or child when a mother is sick.

Where there is no top soil, there is no support system for higher life forms. One hundred and fifty tonnes is the weight of a 2-cm-thick layer in one hectare, which without human or animal intervention would take hundreds of years to develop. But when we and animals intervene to generate and exploit top soil, we can produce massive layers in a relatively short time. This is not always the clean soil we need, however, and we must acknowledge its use to us and our responsibility to it.

One approach to cleaning up the soil and water and keeping ourselves healthy is to recycle organic matter and avoid the use of poisons. Even if you are not fortunate

enough to live in a community that promotes diligent
sorting and recycling, the composting of organic wastes to
promote healthy soil and clean food can be easily managed
on an individual basis. So let's make compost part of the
earth's maintenance diet.

COMPOSTING

Compost bins are vegetarians, although many minute
and not so small life forms live in them. The first stage
of decomposition of organic waste takes place by the
interaction of air, water, microbes and heat. This starts
the breakdown of nitrogen and carbon materials to make
humus, which then becomes food for large and small
organisms in the compost heap. So long as there is humus,
there are organisms feeding off it and making plant
nutrients. Even when the compost has been spread as a
soil additive, micro-organisms remain in it, keeping it
healthy; after we have harvested the crop, they remain
ready to take in more compost with which the depleted
soil should be renewed.

Some of the most easily recognised inhabitants of the
compost heap are the reddish and lumpy brandling worms.
They are not found in garden top soil, for they work
directly on the soft vegetable matter. And for this to
happen it must be collected in a warm, moist
environment, like the centre of a compost heap. Then vast
numbers come up from somewhere deep in the ground.
Alone in a bin with kitchen waste, kept in a warm place,
they will make a rich soil that is more a fertiliser than a
growing medium. In the compost heap, where there is also
woody, fibrous material to be broken down, the end
product has a different composition and is the result of a
complicated team effort. It is the dark, odourless, friable

tilth we call 'gardeners' gold', or compost — Mother Earth's favourite meal.

The results of many trials are available to show the greater capacity of composted soil to germinate seeds as compared with untreated soil; they also show how plants raised on composted soil give greater yields and are more disease-resistant. The HDRA is a good source of information, as is *Composting, An Introduction to the Rational Use of Organic Waste*, by A. Pfirter, A. Von Hirschheydt, P. Ott and H. Vogtmann.

These trial results illustrate that not only is it wasteful of resources and short-term thinking, but it is also criminal to continue to apply artificial fertilisers and pesticides when plants thrive, untreated, in composted soil. Healthy soil is host to the predators of crop pests, and the vigorous plants that composted soil produces are less prone to disease. When poisons are no longer applied to crops, the earth will start to heal — and so, therefore, will we.

Six Sorts of Composting

Field-sheet composting This is a farmers' technique. The residue of a food crop, such as sweet corn or cabbage, is left on the soil surface after the crop has been harvested. It breaks down partially by exposure to weather and is then ploughed into the top soil.

Silage Another farming technique. A crop of 'green manure' is harvested while sappy and fresh, and buried or tightly wrapped. The material is subject to a non-aerobic composting.

Field windrows A farmers' or park-keepers' technique. The wastes from harvesting or pruning are stacked up in heaps or rows and periodically turned, or added to. Roughly hacked, coarse material is used, so the result is a coarse humus which is best laid on the top soil to protect it during winter rains. It is also very effective when laid around the base of plants that are subject to suffering during drought. In both cases, the composted material stays on the surface and is not worked in. It is integrated into the top soil very slowly, which is why it is a useful shield.

Compost heap or bin A gardeners' technique. Hacked autumn and spring prunings are mixed with soft sappy material, such as kitchen vegetable waste and discarded garden plants. The heap is added to at irregular intervals, and varying quantities of materials are added as top-ups.

Compost tumbler or tub Also a gardeners' technique. This is similar to the compost heap, but on a smaller scale, and the hacked material is contained in an enclosed bin that is either rotated or has the contents stirred at regular intervals. Because the smaller volume of material does not generate any heat, the decomposition process must be aided by insulation and human intervention.

Worm bin The non-gardeners' technique. A diagram and building instructions are available from the HDRA. A container with a lid houses the brandling worms on a layer of coarse sand, and they are fed with kitchen vegetable wastes. These then turn into a rich fertiliser/compost which is scooped out of the bin. Because the worms don't like frost, the bin should be kept in a shed, cellar or stair-well. The yield is small, but its quality compensates for the lack of quantity. It makes a great fertiliser for house plants.

Kitchen and garden wastes not processed by the household are collected in Bio-Bins by conscientious councils, but if these are not available, give these wastes to a friend or neighbour who does compost their waste — there's always a shortage of material.

WHAT GOES INTO THE COMPOST BIN?

Any clean vegetable matter, but not roadside plants, because these may be contaminated with heavy metals from motor exhausts. The only animal products that can be processed are feathers and manure. Products such as blood, fishmeal and bonemeal are well-known fertilisers; these are usually worked into the top soil in very small quantities, even if the soil contains compost. Paper in small quantities is all right, as long as it has no printing ink on it (the ink contains toxins). Cooked vegetable material can be included, but avoid any mixed with dairy products. These are almost always oily, and oils block the ventilation of the mass.

Some big fruit stones like those from mangoes or avocados take years to break down. So do nuts in their shells. Both can start sprouting in the soil long after they have been applied to the compost. All material should be seed-free. Try to remove all ripe seed heads; if this is not possible, don't include the plant. All material should be disease-free, and if firm and woody, it should be chopped. A hacker is a good investment. They aren't cheap, but you may be able to work as a cooperative, sharing the cost with a group. Material that is very wet will not go through the hacker, but wet materials can be put directly into the compost heap (which in any case should always be kept moist).

Special additives, such as seaweed and wood ash, are very beneficial in small quantities. Very large quantities of grass-cuttings should be separated into small batches. While they are a good material, to dump them in from the mower bin could stifle the mass when they start to 'mush', which happens very quickly. Yarrow, comfrey and nettles, on the other hand, can go on in in batches — the bigger the better.

Evergreens, even finely hacked, don't break down well (as the name suggests); conifers also contain a pungent resin, which is not beneficial to the compost mass. Autumn leaves gathered into large heaps are best left to rot down on their own, and make a marvellous humus called leaf mould. Despite its name, it is not mouldy; on the contrary, it's another form of 'gardeners' gold'. But if only small amounts are available, they go into the compost bin.

What does Compost have to do with Recycling?

Site your compost bin or pile where you don't have to look at it all the time, but where you can still reach it easily. You will be gathering up all vegetable wastes and trimmings and collecting to keep the pile fed. The whole environment will improve before you have even applied any compost to the soil. The compost bin is just a surround or retaining wall for a compost pile; neither has a base, because the brandling worms must come up into the pile from the ground when the pile first 'appears'; then they disperse once the soft material is processed. The ratio should be twenty-five or thirty times more woody, fibrous matter than green, soft material. This breaks down to 15:1 carbon to nitrogen in the final product, which is considered the ideal ratio. To achieve a good rate of decomposition, the volume of material is important; it is best to gather unmixed materials in some bulk before layering them in a pile. In two or three days, the volume will have reduced dramatically, and if you pull the unchanged materials from the sides into the middle, this will generate another heating up.

Your pile should have started with a mass of at least 1.5 cubic metres. Less volume than this will not heat up.

Obviously, warmer weather helps the process, and in colder regions it is advisable to have solid walls to the bin but still allow air into the mass by turning it regularly. Keep heavy rainfall out of the pile. The material is ready to be applied to the top soil when it has become the texture of soil; if some rough bits remain, sieve them out or leave them in — it depends on your gardening needs.

WHY GO TO SUCH TROUBLE?

Because the alternative is killing us. Yes, for composting you need material, space, time and patience. And for the community collections you need good civic organisation. But the material is free, and if we tidy up a bit, the space is there. Only time is short. Too many of us are already suffering with everything from allergies to cancer; the news is nearly always resonant with the latest environmentally related health scare, which is the result of too little awareness of the organic world. We should stop *thinking* about it and *demand* organically grown food. With solidarity, we could — like a compost heap — become a critical mass; then we could use the energy it takes to attend to our ailments and illnesses to generate change. We must all recognise that we have been sick long enough, and that much of this sickness is a result of what we've done to Mother Earth.

Chapter Eight

Nutritional Therapy as Preventative Medicine

MONICA

Fourteen years ago, a decision was taken which was to have repercussions for everyone across the world. It was the beginning of a study called MONICA (Multinational Monitoring of Trends and Determinants in Cardiovascular Disease), which was undertaken by the World Health Organization. It has been the most ambitious study ever across the nations on the health of people's hearts and circulatory systems. It encompassed the continents, from Australia, through Europe, to Ireland. The cost was an enormous $32 million, and more than ten million men and women were involved in thirty-nine population centres.

HEART DISEASE IN THE NORTH AND SOUTH

As the results became available, a clear pattern emerged: the further north you live, the more likely you are to die of a heart attack. Take two cities — Belfast in Northern Ireland and Toulouse in southern France. The heart disease rate per 100,000 population in Belfast (in the age group forty-five to fifty-four) is 237; in Toulouse, it is 56 per 100,000. In the age group fifty-five to sixty-four, the contrast is even greater — 761 per 100,000 in Belfast, 175 in Toulouse.

Why is there such a remarkable contrast between living in the north and the south? Why should people living in the industrially developed north, with all its wealth, suffer such a high rate of death from heart and vascular disease? What are the protective factors, obviously missing from the northern climes, that are to be found in the south? These questions became even more puzzling, because MONICA studies showed no significant differences in cholesterol, blood pressure, smoking (the three classic indications for heart disease developing) in the countries studied. The further the investigations progress, however, the more clearly we are seeing our answers. Part of the modern world has forgotten the culture of traditional eating. It is clear that southern Europeans know something about diet that the northern peoples have forgotten — or, at least, are no longer practising.

THE EXAMPLE OF FRANCE

For thirty years, Dr Serge Renaud, the French epidemiologist and director of Nutritional Studies at France's National Institute of Health and Medical Research, had been studying the effects of food on his own people in France. The MONICA figures showed that heart disease was highest in countries such as Ireland and Scotland on the one hand, and Australia and the USA on the other, while France was at the bottom. France was bettered only by the Japanese traditional diet of rice, eaten with fish, vegetables, sea vegetables and meat.

The French have a similar blood pressure and cholesterol count as those in the USA, but they outlive the Americans by four years or more, suffer less than half the number of heart attacks, and yet smoke and drink more. This became known as the 'French Paradox'. Dr Renaud was called out of the anonymity of his work to shed light on the puzzle. This he did through a five-year study, completed in 1993, which proved to be a showpiece for the influence of food and eating patterns on health.

Renaud demonstrated his research by taking 600 people who already had cardiac problems and were on a medically recommended diet for heart attacks. He put 300 of these on his own dietary programme; the other 300 remained on their own diet. After five years, the results of the study showed a seventy-six per cent decrease in the chances of a second heart attack for those following Renaud's dietary guidelines. This confirmed the results of his thirty years of work in the field, and the MONICA report.

In addition, it coincided with, and confirmed, the results of the EPIC report (European Prospective Investigation into Cancer and Nutrition), also published in 1993. The population of the northern countries is at greater risk of getting cancer than that of the southern countries. Luxembourg and Belgium lead the mortality figures for men, Denmark and the UK for women. Greece, Portugal and Spain are at the bottom.

DIFFERENCES IN DIET

The helpful foods are as follows: vegetables — fresh, dried or frozen; grains — including bread, pasta, wheat germ, whole brown rice, couscous, bulgar wheat; fruit; low-fat vegetarian cheeses; yoghurt; cottage cheese, etc.; small amounts of oil, olive oil (cold-pressed, virgin); small amounts of low-fat spread; fish; and white meat.

By contrast, unhelpful foods likely to be detrimental to health are: fatty and processed meat; meat preserved with nitrate salt and sugar; battery produced meat; battery produced chicken; battery produced eggs; hard fats — lard, suet, meat drippings; and full-fat cream, cheese and yoghurt (especially when pasteurised and processed with other additives).

In 1993, a major international conference on the
subject of nutrition and public health, called Diets of the
Mediterranean, was held in Cambridge, Massachusetts.
It was remarkable for at least two reasons. Present at the
conference was Ancel Keyes, aged eighty-eight, a man
in robust good health whose message of forty years
previously had been rejected. A great pioneer of modern
nutrition, Keyes was the first person to demonstrate the
relationship between food intake and heart disease.

In his study, which took place in Naples in the 1950s,
Keyes had observed that the wealthy population ate more
butter, milk and red meat, and that they had much higher
rates of death from heart disease than the less well off. The
Neapolitan people made great use of vegetables, fruit,
pasta and bread. They ate little meat, used olive oil instead
of butter and drank wine rather than milk.

Keyes carried out further research in Greece, where
he became convinced that the healthiest diet resembled
what the people of the Mediterranean had been eating for
thousands of years. His intuitive correlation of information
has now been scientifically confirmed. A high-fibre diet,
with plenty of vitamins, minerals, enzymes, essential fats,
natural sugars — and moderation — offers protection
against disease of the circulatory system.

Only four years ago, Dr Martijn Katan, director of the
Department of Human Nutrition at Wageningen
University in Holland, made another brilliant discovery.
Hard margarines — accepted for years as a healthy
substitute for butter — were just as unhealthy, but for an
entirely different reason. Katan discovered that
hydrogenation, the process which converts liquid vegetable
oil to solid or semi-solid spreads, creates trans-fatty acids,
which raise the level of LDLs (low-density lipids —

regarded as bad cholesterol), and leads to clogging of the arteries.

The results of EPIC are now being fully explored. According to Dr Elis Riboli, head of the nutrition and cancer programme at the International Agency for Research on Cancer, we are now seeing that what is bad for cardiovascular disease is bad for cancer. A diet which is rich in fresh fruit and vegetables reduces the risk of most forms of cancer by fifty per cent or more.

CLASSIC DIETS OF THE WORLD
MEXICAN / MEDITERRANEAN / BALKAN
The Solanaceae Family
Tomatoes and aubergines

The Capsicum Family
All peppers

The Cucurbitaceae Family
Zucchini and all squashes

Mediterranean cuisine is rich in grains, legumes, fresh fruits and vegetables. Grain and legumes are a terrific source of fibre, which may protect against colon cancer. Fresh fruit and vegetables are loaded with fibre, as well as beta carotene, vitamin C and other important plant chemicals that may protect against heart disease and cancer.

The Mediterranean diet is short on processed foods, which may be packed with preservatives and saturated fat, and stripped of fibre and nutrients. Meat which is loaded with fat is used sparingly. Eggplant (aubergine), tomato, pepper, garlic and onions are dietary staples; these are all foods that are currently being investigated by the National Cancer Institute for potential cancer-fighting properties.

The Mediterranean diet also calls for an abundance of herbs and spices, such as rosemary, sage, thyme and cumin. Many of these herbs and spices are potent antioxidants, which may protect against atherosclerosis by preventing the oxidation of LDL cholesterol, which is believed to be a major factor in the formation of plaque (plaque deposits on the arterial wall can prevent the flow of blood to vital organs, including the heart).

In many Mediterranean countries, dinner is washed down with a glass of red wine. Red wine contains resveratol, a substance that appears to lower cholesterol. For further information, see *Food as Medicine*, by Earl Mindell.

THE JAPANESE AND MARITIME DIET

These diets have the highest intake of marine or Omega 6 fatty acids. These are even better than the terrestrial-based Omega 3 fatty acids in nuts and seeds. Also eaten are mushrooms and algae (seaweed); green tea is drunk.

THE CHINESE AND KOREAN DIET

In this diet, many stock-based dishes, containing mostly liquid with rice and a little meat (which has been de-fatted by being boiled), are typical. Also eaten are fresh sprouts. The stocks themselves are infusions of herbal roots: ginger, galangal, lemon grass, ginseng and liquorice. As in Japan, green tea is drunk.

See Appendix One for further information on herbs, vitamins, minerals and the properties of foods.

Chapter Nine

Case Studies

Case One
Mary

Mary is a twenty-five-year-old woman. She has eaten a
very poor diet since she became a teenager — and 'always
got away with it', she says. Since Christmas of this year,
she has had spells of extreme pain, shooting from
underneath her front lowest rib, right down her hip,
through to the right of her back and up into the middle
of her back. This pain is always accompanied by nausea,
weakness, complete loss of appetite, and thirst. Her doctor
diagnosed a gallstone, following tests.

Diet

Mary eats nothing for breakfast, and does not even drink
any water. At 10.00 am, for her work break, she has strong
coffee with milk and a few biscuits. For lunch at 1.00 pm,
she has chips, a bar of chocolate and coffee. During her
4.00 pm work break, Mary has more strong coffee and
biscuits. At tea time, she eats take-away pizza, or Chinese
food; in the evening, she has coffee and crisps.

This 'diet' consisted of very little besides fat and
caffeine. There is no fibre worth mentioning, no liquids,
no vegetables, no fruit, no grains, virtually no protein and
plenty of salt and sugar, although they are hidden in the
fast foods and biscuits.

General State of Health

Mary takes no exercise, due to chronic tiredness. Her back
was giving continuous pain. Her breathing capacity was very

poor, due to smoking. The personal history questionnaire she filled in showed a digestive system problem and a very poorly functioning bowel — due in part to the poor diet, and to the sluggish state of her liver and gall bladder.

OBSERVATIONS

A very interesting correlation between the times of the bouts of the severest pain and Mary's diet was confirmed by looking at the calendar: Christmas, New Year, Easter, bank holidays and birthdays. Mary readily admitted to drinking and eating lots more coffee, more refined foods and alcohol on all of these occasions.

TREATMENT PROGRAMME

Because Mary had come along at the request of her concerned boyfriend — who is very health-conscious and recognises that Mary has an addiction to caffeine — I then asked her permission to set out a nutrition programme. Would she feel ready to take full responsibility for her own health? Would she be prepared to make more effort to apply the principles of the 'four doctors':

- sun/air
- exercise/rest
- good food
- good water.

Mary's answer was: 'I am prepared to do anything that is necessary.'

I drew three charts for her, which were to go up on the refrigerator door. Every day, Mary is to remind herself about the stress-sugar cycle, and the body clock for eating times. When she learns to stay within the framework of both, she will regain control over her life. These three charts became Mary's guidelines.

THE BODY'S BIOLOGICAL EATING CLOCK

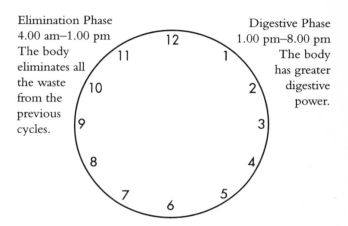

Elimination Phase
4.00 am–1.00 pm
The body eliminates all the waste from the previous cycles.

Digestive Phase
1.00 pm–8.00 pm
The body has greater digestive power.

Assimilation Phase
1.00 am–4.00 am
The body has a full-time job of assimilation of food.

LOW BLOOD SUGAR CLOCK

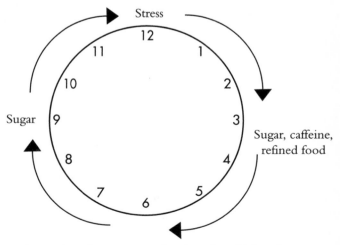

Stress

Sugar, caffeine, refined food

Sugar

The result is that your mood swings from high to low, anxiety, depression, poor energy levels.

LOW BLOOD SUGAR CORRECTION CLOCK

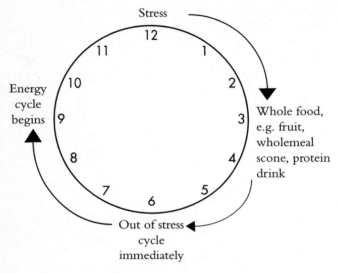

Stress

Energy cycle begins

Whole food, e.g. fruit, wholemeal scone, protein drink

Out of stress cycle immediately

There is an even release of energy for hours, mood normal, with a sense of well-being.

My nutritional advice to Mary was as follows below.

Begin the day with a large glass of warm water. Take one teaspoon of olive oil (virgin olive oil, first pressing) to help the digestion. For breakfast, have an apple, pear, peach *or* a handful of grapes; a slice of wholemeal bread, with sugar-free jam *or* marmalade; and a cup of camomile or peppermint tea. Both these teas are good digestive aids, calming, soothing, allowing the working of the digestive system in such a way that the person feels lighter and brighter. A cup of light tea, *or* herbal coffee, at work. If she felt the need for a cup of real coffee, she was to make it weaker than usual. Lunch was to be: brown bread, *or* scone; fish *or* chicken *or* turkey; natural yoghurt; and fresh fruit. Dinner gave Mary quite a lot of scope: vegetables in great variety, with rice, *or* pasta, *or* potato; fish *or* vegetarian tofu, *or* risotto, *or* vegetable and rice stir-fry, *or* vegetable lasagne, *or* shell pasta with tuna, onion, parsley and a little good-quality oil. (All pasta, rice and grains to be wholemeal.)

Mary has decided to wean herself off coffee over a six- to eight-week time span, by slow reduction, and by introducing a range of simple herbal teas.

SHORT-TERM OUTCOME

After one month on this programme — greatly helped by her boyfriend and her mother — Mary had a list of small but significant improvements. Her pain had eased within one week. In fact, she observed that after eating her meals according to the plan, she experienced freedom from acid indigestion, belching and bad breath. She was aware of her improved hair and skin — which had been blotchy, with angry red patches at times — due to all the good food, and plenty of water. Mary's energy levels were slightly better; while she missed the caffeine, Mary realised that she was on a much more even keel mood-wise than previously. She now had regular visits to the toilet, instead of her previous irregular pattern (perhaps only once every three days).

Mary is enjoying the new wide way of looking at food, with better variety in all her meals. Looking at her charts helped her to make out a shopping list, and she also avoided shopping when feeling very hungry.

RETURN VISIT

Kinesiology testing on this visit suggested that her stone was now more gravelly; in fact, it seemed to be dissolving. This was due to the effect of the pectin in the fruits, the olive oil in her diet (taken on a daily basis), all the vitamin-A rich vegetables, the plentiful supply of water, brown bread and the herbal teas. Kinesiology is a system of biofeedback from the body, using muscle testing. It is based on the principle that certain muscle groups are related to specific parts of the body. Such tests are used to detect and rectify energy blockages and any imbalances which cause illness. The practitioner uses light touch and deep massage, and gives dietary advice.

A big bonus was that her back now felt much stronger, due to the mineral-rich foods being absorbed into the bloodstream.

The only supplement added to her programme was aloe vera organic, in order gently to encourage improvements in the entire digestive system. Her eating programme remains the same, although she is encouraged to shop for wider varieties of all types of foods on her menu. Special foods for Mary included the following: apples; apple juice; artichokes; beetroot; beetroot juice; carrots; carrot juice; cranberries; sugar-free cranberry juice; dandelion instead of lettuce; dandelion tea *or* coffee; garlic; grapefruit (pink); olives (unsalted); parsley; parsley tea; pears; red radish; white radish (mooli); water (pure).

LONG-TERM OUTCOME

What began as a gallstone for Mary became at the end of her treatment programme a small amount of broken stone (gravel), which the body can further break down and discharge slowly. This is as a result of the nutrients and diet Mary was on. This is the process of cleaning the liver and gall-bladder naturally. Follow-up treatment will continue to use very gentle, effective herbal tonics to maintain Mary's general health and continue the process of breaking down the stone. In all cases such as Mary's, we ask the patient's doctor to monitor his or her progress.

Under the supervision of her doctor, Mary has continued to become healthier, with a renewed interest in her own ability to have beautiful skin, hair, nails, teeth and bones. She has a healthy appetite, good energy and is pain-free — all her systems are 'go'.

CASE TWO
JEAN

Jean remembered being a hyperactive twelve-year-old. The diet which was recommended for her did not help, and she had been off dairy products at the time; there was no beneficial result. She has recently married.

DIET

Jean and her husband Manuel live in a country area, and grow a great selection of vegetables, including salad vegetables through the summer months. They have free-range eggs from their hens, and a good, pure water system.

GENERAL STATE OF HEALTH

Jean's stress levels had climbed above the normal for many reasons. At first, she felt irritable, hyperactive and distressed. She then began to have symptoms of bowel distress and menstrual cycle problems. Every morning when she rose from bed, she would have diarrhoea. She was referred to a specialist by her doctor. After a large number of tests, she was diagnosed as having a hyperactive thyroid gland, and she began treatment, with a high dose of neo-mercazole. She began to respond after one month of this treatment.

SYMPTOMS

Some of the symptoms of hyperthyroidism, or
thyrotoxicosis, are: feeling too hot even when the
temperature is cool; a great feeling of needing air, due to an
increased need for oxygen by the body; heart palpitations,
or disturbed rhythm; excessive energy; poor sleep; and
severe weight loss. It can affect men and women. In
women, disturbance of the menstrual cycle can occur.
Occasionally, there can be protrusion of the eyes. Jean had
symptoms of weight loss, heart rhythm irregularity,
apprehension and anxiety as a result of her condition.

TREATMENT PROGRAMME

Jean decided, with permission from her doctor, to work
with a programme of lifestyle and dietary adjustments,
together with counselling. Studying Louise Hay's positive
approaches to handling very difficult emotions became an
important support throughout the programme. Jean made
an appointment to see the nutritional counsellor.

On her first visit to her nutritionist, Jean made a list
of very positive changes to her diet. Each day, she would
include some organic grains, including: millet, brown rice,
whole oats, buckwheat, cornmeal (maize), quinoa and
wheat for wholemeal bread and pasta.

A special emphasis was placed on the following foods:
aduki beans; butter beans; dried fruit with sweet rice and
millet; ginger; garlic; green vegetables (broccoli, kale,
cabbage, sprouts); miso soup; protein drink (dairy-, egg-,
sugar- and yeast-free); rice *or* buckwheat noodles; root
vegetables (carrots, turnips, parsnips); and stewed fruit.
The ginger and garlic were to improve the circulation and
the appetite, and to calm the digestive system. Food
supplements to help her digestion included acidophilus,

and kelp powder, or tablets, in very small amounts. Special herbs were included in order to cleanse and heal the bowel, along with B-complex vitamins.

All the foods listed in Jean's menu have calming, centring, soothing and comforting properties. She consciously chose foods free from additives, residues or processing because her body would then not have to compete to receive its nutrients. She enjoyed her own eggs and made lots of salads in the summer. Fish and white meat were added to the diet as good sources of essential fats and protein.

REBUILDING THE BODY

Because Jean had lost a lot of weight, and consequently minerals, vitamins, enzymes and essential fats, it was absolutely vital to include top-quality supplements in her programme. Jean became very intuitive about the needs of her own body. At her consultations, she discussed how she was feeling both physically and emotionally. She related how very helpful she found the protein drink, which staved off the sinking feeling she used to have between meals. It also gave her sufficient energy to prepare her next meal.

Jean's requirements for essential fats (CFA) were very great. Her previous eating habits had not included sufficient sources. Now her hormonal and nervous systems were causing concern. Evening primrose oil was added to the programme, in order to begin the process of healing. Fatty acids are the foundations and the protectors of a strong, healthy nervous system. As folic acid and vitamin B12 are two of the cooperating workers involved in the synthesis of essential fats, the evening primrose was taken at the same time as the protein drink, which contained both. As she

became more skilled in the management of her shopping
and preparation of foods, Jean tried new sources of
essential fats, which also happened to be calcium- and
magnesium-rich.

NEW FOODS

Jean then integrated a variety of new foods into her diet,
including: almonds (toasted, and ground in a coffee
grinder); dillisk *or* dulse *or* wakame (all rich sources of
minerals, including calcium and iron, and also fats); feta
cheese; sea vegetables, e.g. kombu (added to soups,
casseroles and vegetable dishes); sunflower seeds; tahini
(sesame seed spread); tofu; and vegetarian cheese.

SAMPLE LUNCH MENU

One pitta bread, toasted to pop open, with various fillings,
including: shredded lettuce, chopped chives, feta cheese,
small tomato *or* a little red pepper, one teaspoon olive oil,
chopped basil. Mix the filling together. Open up the pitta
bread, fill with mixture, decorate with watercress, cress. In
winter, a hot bowl of a soup such as minute soup to begin
the meal; in summer natural yoghurt after the meal.

A recipe for minute soup is as follows. Liquidise one
mug of lightly cooked carrots and one mug of cooked,
diced potatoes. Add two mugs of vegetable juice from
previously cooked vegetables, *or* add pure unsweetened
carrot juice (Biotta brand, if available). Heat through —
do not boil. Decorate with parsley and sage.

COUNSELLING

During the year, Jean began to receive counselling, which
she found of immense help in settling her emotions. Her
priorities gradually changed from very, very high

expectations of perfection from herself to more achievable goals. Belief systems she had held for a long time were revealed and replaced with new, positive thought patterns.

OUTCOME

The effects of the chosen foods could be seen over the next few months. Jean gradually found herself becoming less overwhelmed, less impatient, less tense and hyperactive. She also noticed herself being more and more satisfied with her meals, and correctly concluded that this was due to the increasing efficiency of her digestion.

Jean also began a course in theatre development. This included learning to discover the child within. This was a turning point in her life, and Jean's happiness was wonderful to see. Her eyes had a new light, her appetite improved and she began to put back on the lost weight. All diarrhoea stopped. Her menstrual cycle became normal, and her nervous system became calm. Now she wanted to achieve her greatest desire — to have a child.

Her specialist reduced the neo-mercazole very slowly to the minimum dose. Her nutrition was changed to pre-pregnancy vitamins and minerals and folic acid. Within six weeks, the happy news was that Jean and Manuel were expecting their first child. Jean's health was exceptional throughout the pregnancy. Their baby girl arrived safe and sound. It can be said that due — at least in part — to the wonderful nutritional regime followed by both parents (Manuel ate the same food as Jean), the baby had a gentle, swift entry into the world.

The baby is healthy, calm and good-humoured. Needless to say, Jean is extremely pleased with her new way of eating. She feels it was worth all the effort she made at the very start of her programme to become a skilled cook of natural, whole, unprocessed foods. The benefits are to be seen in each family member.

CASE THREE
MARK

Twelve-year-old Mark was referred to me for kinesiology, allergy tests and nutrition by a remarkable priest, who also has the gift of healing. The priest felt that Mark was in need not only of spiritual but also of nutritional help. Mark's case illustrates very well the way in which holistic healing recognises that the person is a spiritual as well as physical being, and that all the individual's aspects — mental, emotional and physical — may need to be addressed in the process of healing. Mark's ambition was to be a top–class footballer, although his lack of energy was severely restricting the amount of football and other games he could play.

DIET
Mark's diet was high in dairy foods.

GENERAL STATE OF HEALTH
Mark was underweight for his age, completely lacking in energy and suffering from severe bouts of asthma. He was missing a lot of school, and was emotionally upset at times. There was no family history of any degenerative diseases — although previous generations had had poor circulation and respiratory problems — and until recently there had been no cancer in the family. His parents, strong people who had previously both been well, were suffering from stress and general ill health.

KINESIOLOGY AND NUTRITIONAL TESTS
The kinesiology tests showed Mark to be living in a house with high levels of electromagnetic energy and geopathic

stress (i.e. watr under the ground which disturbs the function of the human body). Both can be caused by electrical equipment, such as microwaves, pylons outside the home, underground water and radon gas.

The nutritional tests found that Mark was very undernourished, due to a weak and poorly functioning thyroid gland, which in turn affected his metabolism. This was the cause of his sluggishness and the fact that he felt cold even in warm rooms. His allergy test showed that certain foods he was regularly eating were not agreeing with him, and were causing all other good foods to be blocked in their absorption.

The highest allergy foods were: all dairy products, yeast, beet sugar, monosodium glutamate, additives, chemicals, colourings, preservatives, red E102 tartrazine, yellow E104 quinoline, yellow E110, E120 cochineal, E122 carmoisine, E123 amaranth, E124 ponceau, E127 erythrisine, E128 and red 126. All of these can be triggers for hyperactive behaviour, asthma, urticaria, gastric stomach, insomnia and vomiting.

Treatment Programme

We discussed the environment, the allergies and a new dietary approach that would, over the next two months, exclude the known allergic foods.

Mark's parents were advised to switch off as much of their electrical equipment as possible and to allow a very limited amount of television. Other measures included moving Mark into a spare bedroom that was further away from electrical equipment such as fuse boxes, video recorders and the television; children are a great deal more sensitive to electromagnetic waves than adults.

Mark's nutritional programme included a gradual move onto goat's milk, yoghurt and cheese. Extra supplies of foods that benefit the respiratory system had to be included in Mark's diet, such as: chicken broth (contains an anti-inflammatory); garlic; green vegetable soups; home-made barley and lemon water; lemons; lentil, chickpea *or* split pea soup. A good, nourishing, hot breakfast every morning was important — whole grain bread, porridge oats, home-made pancakes, scrambled eggs on toast, potatoes and rice made into burger or sausage shapes and grilled or fried in good-quality oil, potato cakes with spaghetti made from buckwheat, corn or rice.

For lunch, Mark was to have hot soup and a salad sandwich made with rye, oat or wholemeal bread. Dinner should include two vegetables (one green); whole grain rice, buckwheat, corn, *or* millet *or* potato; with one of the following: chicken, fish, lamb, turkey, vegetarian risotto, vegetarian *or* lamb lasagne, *or* vegetable casserole. For dessert, Mark was to eat home-made apple pie, apple *or* rhubarb crumble, apple strudel, natural yoghurt.

It was important to add lots of parsley, onion, garlic, thyme and horseradish to the foods. Liquids should include hot lemon, barley and honey drinks, to clear the mucous congestion from the respiratory system. Recommended supplements were:

- aromatherapy oil of cajuput in a very high dilution, with almond oil (for massaging the chest and lungs every morning and evening)
- Bach flower remedies (specially chosen to strengthen, encourage and motivate Mark to get better)
- cod liver oil
- evening primrose oil

- garlic capsules
- vitamin C (buffered, i.e. non-acid, more easily tolerated by delicate stomachs).

OUTCOME

Over a period of two months, the treatment programme brought about a remarkable degree of recovery, and Mark is still in touch two years later. He is continuing to go from strength to strength. Mark's mother had his complete cooperation from the very outset of his treatment; she explained everything about his diet and lifestyle that she was changing, and asked him for feedback. His appetite became good, and he enjoyed all his food and was willing to try new ones. He gained weight, slept very well, and was able to fight off any threat of a cold, cough or infection which might start up the asthma again. Mark has also noticed a greater tolerance of weather changes. His doctor has monitored his doses of asthma medicine throughout, gradually reducing the prescription as needed.

Finally, Mark is progressing very well in physical sports, particularly football.

FURTHER RECOMMENDATIONS

In winter, the elderberry fruit was recommended as a regular part of Mark's prevention regime. Made into a hot drink with peppermint tea and honey, it will act powerfully against catarrh and inflammation; it is also rich in vitamin C — and it is in any case delicious! Suggestions that have proven helpful in the steady and continuing healing of Mark's lungs have been: reflexology, deep breathing exercises and maintaining a good posture. Good posture was emphasised because those with lung problems tend to hunch their shoulders and develop a round shoulder posture, which is very unhealthy.

CASE FOUR
ROBERT

Robert, a five-year-old boy with Down's syndrome, came to see me, brought by his mother.

DIET

His favourite foods, of which Robert ate a lot, were sweet buns and biscuits, cheddar cheese sandwiches, fromage frais and ice cream.

GENERAL STATE OF HEALTH

Robert's biggest problem is his susceptibility to colds, which go straight down to his chest, becoming a constant cough which nothing seems to clear. He also produces a mucous discharge from his nose.

TREATMENT PROGRAMME

Robert's mother and I discussed at length how best to rearrange his diet, in order to incorporate less of the above foods and more fruit and vegetables. We agreed that she would slowly, over a period of two months, make the necessary changes to Robert's diet.

My suggestions were as follows: for breakfast three mornings a week, Robert was to have baby oat flakes porridge with honey and a little milk; two mornings a week, he was to have a high-fibre, low-sugar (raw sugar) cereal, with juice or milk; on the remaining two mornings, he would have an egg or beans on brown, wholemeal toast.

Mid-morning, Robert could have fresh fruit in season, and a drink of water. Lunch would consist of a bowl of carrot and potato soup, *or* chicken broth, *or* vegetable soup (mainly green vegetables, with added parsley and onions), *or* lentil soup; with wholemeal brown bread scones, *or* rice cakes, *or* rye bread, *or* oat cakes with tahini spread, *or* almond nut butter, *or* sunflower butter.

His mid-afternoon snack would be fresh fruit in season (e.g. mashed banana) with a dairy-free ice cream, such as soya ice cream. For dinner, Robert could have a puréed (instead of chopped) selection of vegetables; with potatoes, rice *or* whole grain pasta; and fish, turkey, chicken *or* lamb; dessert was to be natural yoghurt and a slice of carrot cake. (Vegetable purée is far more easily digested and a more valuable source of nutrition for children.)

ADDITIONAL SUGGESTIONS

A selection of Dr Bach flower remedies were made up to help Robert to adjust to the dietary changes and to strengthen his immune system. The aromatherapy oils camomile and lavender were made up in almond oil to massage the little boy's back and chest twice daily, in order to increase circulation, strengthen the lung muscles and build up resistance to infection. The oils were greatly diluted because of Robert's age.

I also suggested that Robert spend less time sitting at television, with instead more walks and sport. I emphasised that small meals were sensible, as little and often at the age of five is very helpful to the developing digestive system, and helps the child not to put on too much weight.

OUTCOME

I have kept in touch with Robert and his mother for over six years. He has become a fine, radiantly healthy young boy, who enjoys his food, school, his friends and family.

CASE FIVE

MAEVE

Maeve is a woman who found difficulty in achieving correct diagnosis or assistance through conventional medical treatment. Her mother's protracted illness in hospital, and subsequent death, had put Maeve under considerable stress. Following conventional treatment for problems with her womb, Maeve found out about alternative medicine, which she then decided to try.

GENERAL STATE OF HEALTH

Maeve had three small operations on her womb in 1994, which needed subsequent treatment with two courses of antibiotics. Her immune system was low, and she had a viral flu that left her so tired that she spent ten days able to do nothing but sit on the couch. On a visit to her GP she was told that nothing could be done for her, and that her exhaustion may have been from ME, a common aftermath of viral flu.

SYMPTOMS

Along with the extreme tiredness, Maeve has a number of other problems. Her stomach and bowel swell up after eating certain foods, and this is accompanied by an uncomfortable, itchy feeling. She has a craving for sweet foods and chocolate, and eating sugar in any food causes her skin to come out in a rash, especially on her back. Her sinuses are also irritated; she becomes breathless just

walking up the stairs and has no energy. Consequently,
her mental state is one of complete despondency.

KINESIOLOGY AND VEGA TESTS
These tests revealed that Maeve had candida albicans — a
yeast infection; she had an intolerance to sugar and yeast;
her immune system was very low; her liver and small
intestine were affected; and she had a chemical allergy.
Maeve was very relieved to discover what the root cause
of her problem was.

Vega testing originated from electro-acupuncture
according to Voll (EAV). It is based on measuring
electrical conductivity by applying an electrode, which
is held by the patient.

TREATMENT PROGRAMME
Maeve began an anti-candida programme straight away,
cutting out all sugar and yeast from her diet and using
supplements. She also used homeopathic anti-fungal drops.
After six weeks, she introduced caprylic acid, which kills
off the candida infection in the body. The reaction to the
treatment meant that Maeve felt somewhat worse for a few
weeks, with flu-like symptoms and pains in her legs.

SHORT-TERM OUTCOME
Having completed this stage of the treatment, Maeve felt
much better, even though she had lost a lot of weight.

ADDITIONAL DIETARY MEASURES
Maeve then began to eat garlic, and took cold-pressed virgin
olive oil. She also took the herbal tea pau d'arco, which is
anti-fungal, and drank aloe vera juice. She began to replace
the friendly bacteria in the bowel with a course of

acidophilus. She discovered a wonderful herb, golden seal, which is anti-fungal, antibiotic and in addition boosts the immune system.

A SETBACK

Maeve felt so much better after six months, although still much thinner than she had been before, that she celebrated her new-found energy and health with two vodkas. However, because of her sensitivity to chemicals, this set her back considerably. Having put a strain on her liver with the chemical overload, her intestinal ecology was upset, which encouraged the parasites. Maeve was then treated with grapefruit seed extract. Because her body was not breaking down foods into usable nutrients, she was put on digestive enzymes.

LONG-TERM OUTCOME

It took eighteen months in total for the candida to be cleared out of Maeve's system. She is still careful with her diet and her alcohol intake. It has been a tremendous learning experience for her, and she believes that the over-use of antibiotics and the over-consumption of processed foods are bringing about increasing numbers of cases of candida albicans. Maeve is doing very well, and has begun studying anatomy, physiology and nutrition, with a view to taking a diploma.

APPENDIX ONE

HERBS AND THEIR BENEFITS

Herb	Benefits
Almond	Skin
Aloe vera	Skin
Anise	Digestion
Apple	Digestion, lowers cholesterol
Artichoke	Liver
Basil	Digestion
Bilberry	Eyesight
Borage	Gamma linoleic acid
Calendula	Pain reliever
Camomile	Vitamin C
Capsicum	Vitamin C
Caraway	Digestion
Carrot	Anti-cancer
Cayenne	Soothing
Comfrey	Relieves sores
Cone flower	Anti-urinary tract infection
Cranberry	Liver, gall-bladder
Dandelion	Boosts immune system
Evening primrose	Reduces stress and tension
Fenugreek	Lowers blood sugar levels
Feverfew	Headaches
Garlic	Antibiotic effect, anti-cancer
Ginger	Digestion, calms stomach
Ginkgo	All-round booster
Ginseng	Increases endurance
Golden seal	Skin problems
Horse chestnut	Veins
Juniper berry	Urinary tract infections
Nettle	Lowers blood sugar, iron

Herb	Benefits
Raspberry	Good for women generally
Shiitake mushroom	Boosts immune system
Turmeric	Cleans blood, gall-bladder

FOODS AND THEIR PROPERTIES

Foods	Properties
Garlic, onions, raw carrots, shiitake mushrooms	Anti-cancer
Turmeric, garlic, cayenne and ginkgo	Circulation
Evening primrose, cayenne, garlic, olive oil, oat bran, artichoke	Heart
Echinacea (cone flower)	Immune system booster
Milk thistle, artichoke, dandelion, turmeric	Liver

FOOD SOURCES OF MINERALS

Mineral	Sources
Phosphorus	Alfalfa, avocado, beets, Brussels sprouts, cabbage, coconut, corn, peas
Potassium	Alfalfa, avocado, beans (string), dates, dandelions, greens, parsnips, potato peel

Mineral	Sources
Silicon	Beets, cantaloupe, grains (whole, sprouted), horseradish, horsetail and oat straw tea, parsnips
Sodium	Alfalfa, cabbage, carrots, celery, goat's milk (and whey), lettuce, spinach, watermelon
Sulphur	Alfalfa, avocado, Brussels sprouts, broccoli, cabbage, cranberries, kale, pumpkin, watercress

BOTANICAL VITAMIN SOURCES

Vitamin	Sources
Vitamin A	Alfalfa, annatto, dandelion, watercress, parsley, paprika, kelp
Vitamin B	Apples, bananas, beans, beets, cabbage, carrots, corn, grapefruit, onions, oranges, peas, potatoes, raisins, spinach, tomatoes, wheat, whole seeds, yeast
Vitamin C complex	All greens and citrus fruits
Vitamin C	Annatto, watercress, wheat germ, all oil-containing seeds

Vitamin	Sources
Vitamin D	All seeds, alfalfa, oats, flax, sesame, wheat germ, soya beans, tofin, dulse, kelp, watercress
Vitamin E	Alfalfa, chestnut leaves
Vitamin K	Rose hips, black and red currants, strawberries, potatoes, spinach, cabbage, watercress

FOODS FOR RAPID HEALING

Fruits	Apples, apricots, cherries, dates, figs (fresh or dried), grapefruit, grapes, lemons, oranges, pears, peaches, plums, prunes (dried), raisins, raspberries and strawberries
Vegetables	Asparagus, beans (string), cabbage (raw), carrots (raw), cauliflower (raw), celery (raw), cucumber, garlic, green peppers, lettuce, onions (raw), parsnips, peas, spinach, tomatoes and watercress

E NUMBERS AND THEIR EFFECTS

E102	Tartrazine	Hyperactivity, asthma, blurred vision, skin problems, insomnia
E104, E107,	Quinoline yellow	Hyperactivity, asthma, eczema, insomnia
E120	Cochineal	Hyperactivity, asthma, eczema, insomnia
E110	Sunset yellow	Hyperactivity, asthma, gastric upset, vomiting, urticaria, insomnia
E124	Ponceau	Hyperactivity, asthma, insomnia, possibly cancer
E131	Patent blue	Skin sensitivity, nausea, low blood pressure, breathing problems
E132	Indigo carmine	High blood pressure, hypertension, skin problems, breathing problems
E133, E128, E142	Brilliant blue	Hyperactivity, asthma, insomnia, urticaria
E201, E202, E203	Sodium sorbate	Asthma, skin irritation, hay fever

E221	Sodium sulphite	Asthma, destruction of vitamins E and B1
E210	Benzoic acid	Asthma, gastric irritation, neurological disorders, reacts with E222
E230, E231, E232	Biphenyl	Nausea, vomiting, irritation to eyes and nose
E239	Hexamine	Gastric upsets, gene mutations in animal studies, rashes, cancer
E249	Potassium nitrate	Asthma, destruction of red blood corpuscles, cancer
E250, E251, E252	Sodium nitrate	Dizziness, cancer in animals, deoxygenation of blood

APPENDIX TWO

A Typical Daily Menu

This menu is based on the principle of restoring health; the ingredients have been chosen to stimulate your metabolism, nourish the muscles, and help you stabilise your weight.

Breakfast Swiss muesli, based on: oat flakes, or millet flakes, with chopped apricots (steeped overnight in water), *or* almonds, *or* a little pear, apple *or* berries, blueberries, blackberries, blackcurrants; tea (low caffeine); wholemeal, rye *or* wheat bread; almond *or* tahini spread, sugar-free marmalade *or* sugar-free fruit spread.

Lunch Vegetable soup *or* home-made soup made from any meat, *or* some chicken *or* fish; baked potato with coleslaw *or* cottage cheese with herbs (parsley, watercress, horseradish, garlic); a small salad in winter, a large salad in summer, including as many available grains and vegetables as you like.

Dinner Try to eat an early meal, with plenty of time to enjoy and digest it before retiring. Eat traditional dishes, such as casserole of vegetables, and meat, with lentils, chickpeas *or* aduki beans. If you plan ahead, you can cook enough grain for three days. Then combine it with rice, millet *or* whole grain pasta, with a tasty selection of vegetables. Add any meat *or* fish in a very small amount, with soup.

Suggested dinner menu Vegetarian *or* meat lasagne. If you make meat lasagne, halve the meat content by using an equal quantity of red lentils, pre-cooked for twenty minutes (one cup of lentils to two cups water *or* stock).

Vegetarian curry *or* meat curry. Reduce the meat by including extra vegetables, chickpeas *or* Quorn.

Vegetarian nut loaf *or* meat loaf. Again, reduce the quantity of meat by adding one mug of cooked grains.

Stir-fry dish. Try a potato and vegetable selection; simply cut your vegetables up into similar-sized chunks, including the potatoes. Cook potato and onion in olive *or* sunflower oil for six to eight minutes, then add diced red pepper and carrots. Cook for about three minutes until crunchy, then add tomatoes, garlic, parsley, feta cheese, tofu, chicken *or* fish. Put a lid on your wok *or* saucepan. Heat through thoroughly, and serve with salad, rice noodles, wholemeal spaghetti *or* millet. The total preparation and cooking time is only around twenty-five minutes, or less.

Helpful Addresses

IRELAND AND THE UK

Action Against Allergy
24–6 High Street, Hampton Hill, Middlesex TW12 1PD.
Helpful for those with extreme allergy problems,
particularly in tracking down books on the various aspects
of the subject.

Association of Systematic Kinesiology
39 Browns Road, Surbiton, Surrey KT5 8ST.

British Complementary Medicine Association
9 Soar Lane, Leicester LE3 5DE.
Tel.: 0116 242 5406.

**Foresight: The Association for the Promotion of
Pre-Conceptual Care**
Reg. Charity No. 279160.
The Oly Vicarage, Whitley, Godalming, Surrey GU8 5PN.

Henry Doubleday Research Association (HDRA)
Ryton-on-Dunsmore, Coventry CU8 3LG.
Tel.: 01203 303517.

Hyperactivity Association
71 Whyke Lane, Chichester, West Sussex PO19 2LD.
Tel.: 01903 725182.

**Irish Organic Farmers and Growers Association
(IOFGA)**
56 Blessington Street, Dublin 7.
Tel.: 3531 830 7996.
Produces *Irish Consumer Guide to Organic Food*, compiled
by Shirley Cully.

McCarrison Society

24 Paddington Street, London W1M 4DR.

Medic–Alert Foundation

1 Bridge Wharf, 156 Caledonian Road, London N1 9UU.
Tel.: 0171 833 3034.

National Pure Water Association

12 Dennington Lane, Crigglestone, Wakefield WF4 3ET.
Tel.: 01924 254433.
Campaigns to remove the legislation which allows
fluoridation of water.

Society for the Promotion of Nutritional Therapy (SPNT)

PO Box 47, Heathfield, East Sussex TN22 8ZX.
Tel.: 01435 867007.
Send stamped addressed envelope and £1 for information.

Soil Association

86 Colston Street, Bristol BS1 5BB.
Tel.: 0117 929 0661.

Stepping Stones

Sroughan, Lacken, Blessington, Co. Wicklow.
Specialist with Dr Bach's flower remedies.

Working Weekends on Organic Farms (WWOOF)

19 Bradford Road, Lewes, East Sussex BN17 1RB.
Tel.: 01273 476286.

AUSTRALIA AND NEW ZEALAND

Bio-Gro New Zealand

PO Box 9693, Marion Square, Wellington 6031.
Tel.: 644 801 9741.

Brisbane Organic Growers Group
PO Box 236, Lutwyche, Queensland 4030.
Tel.: 617 32771507.

International Kinesiology College
PO Box 25–162, St Heliers, Auckland 1130.
Tel.: 649 575 2818.

International Kinesiology College
PO Box 164, Buderim, Queensland 4556.
Tel.: 617 445429.

Nutritional Foods Association of Australia
PO Box 1075, Chatswood, New South Wales 2067.
Tel.: 612 9411 6348.

Organic Gardening and Farming Society of Tasmania
PO Box 228, Ulverstone, Tasmania 7315.
Tel.: 613 6437 5218.

Organic Growers Association New South Wales
49 South Liverpool Road, Heckenberg, New South Wales 2168.
Tel.: 612 9825 0078.

Science and Computing Department
PO Box 22095, Christchurch Polytechnic, Te Whare Runanga O Otautahi.
Tel.: 643 364 9037.
Runs courses on biological and sustainable food production.

Recommended Reading

Airola, Paavo O., *Health Secrets from Europe*, New York: Arco Publishing 1972.

Barnard, Julian, *Patterns of Life Force*, Hereford: The Bach Educational Programme 1988.

Barnard, Julian and Martine, *The Healing Herbs of Edward Bach*, Hereford: The Bach Educational Programme 1988.

Bircher Benner Clinic, *Bircher Benner Nutrition Plan for Skin Problems*, New York: Pyramid Books 1973.

Blande, Jeffrey, *Your Personal Health*, Northamptonshire: Thorson's 1984.

Carson, Rachel, *Silent Spring*, Penguin Books in association with Hamish Hamilton 1963.

Chelminski, Rudolph, 'A Great Way to Live Longer', in *Reader's Digest*, London: Reader's Digest September 1994.

Clark, Hulda Regehr, *The Cure for All Cancers*, San Diego: ProMotion Publications 1993.

Clark, Hulda Regehr, *The Cure for All Diseases*, San Diego: ProMotion Publications 1995.

Colbin, Annemarie, *Food and Healing*, New York: Ballantine Books 1986.

Costigan, Brenda, *For Goodness Sake*, Dublin: Crescent Press 1992.

Davies, Dr Steven and Stewart, Dr Alan, *A Nutritional Medicine*, London: Pan Books 1987.

De Vries, Jan, *How to Live a Healthy Life*, Edinburgh: Mainstream Press 1995.

De Vries, Jan, *Menopause*, Edinburgh: Mainstream Press 1993.

De Vries, Jan, *Menstrual and Premenstrual Tension*, Edinburgh: Mainstream Press 1992.

De Vries, Jan, *The Miracle of Life*, Edinburgh: Mainstream Press 1987.

De Vries, Jan, *Stomach and Bowel Disorders*, Edinburgh: Mainstream Press 1993.

De Vries, Jan, *Stress and Nervous Disorders*, Edinburgh: Mainstream Press 1994.

De Vries, Jan, *Viruses, Allergies and the Immune System*, Edinburgh: Mainstream Press 1988.

Emsley, John, *The Consumer's Good Chemical Guide*, London: Corgi 1996.

Fathman, George and Doris, *Live Foods*, California: Ehret Literature Publishing 1967.

Flatto, Edwin, *Revitalise your Body with Nature's Secrets*, New York: Arco Publishing 1973.

Grieve, M., *A Modern Herbal*, London: Tiger Books 1973.

Halvorsen, Brian and Flemming, Susan, *The Natural Dentist*, London: Century Arrow 1986.

Hay, Louise, *Empowering Women*, America: Hay House, 1997.

Heinerman, John, *Heinerman's Encyclopedia of Fruits and Vegetables*, New York: Parker 1988.

Houlton, Jane, *The Allergy Survival Guide*, London: Random House 1995.

Jacka, Judy, *Frontiers of Natural Therapies*, Victoria: Lothian 1989.

Kaminski, Patricia and Katz, Richard, *The Flower Essence Repertory*, California: Flower Essence Society 1994.

Katz, Martha Ellen, *High Protein Baking*, New York: Ballantine 1975.

Keane, Mary T., *Health through Wise Living*, Tipperary: Advance Publishing.

Kiester, Edwin and Valente, Sally, 'Little Known Signs of a
     Heart Attack', in *Reader's Digest*, London: Reader's
     Digest August 1993.

Kinderlehrer, Jane, *How to Feel Younger Longer*, New York:
     Rodale 1974.

La Tourelle, Maggie and Courtenay, Anthea, *Thorson's
     Introductory Guide to Kinesiology*, Northamptonshire:
     Thorson's 1992.

Lacey, Richard, *Unfit for Human Consumption, Food in
     Crisis*, London: Grafton 1991.

Lappé, Frances Moore, *Diet for a Small Planet*, New York:
     Ballantine 1971.

Larson, Gena, *Better Food for Better Babies and their Families*,
     Connecticut: Pivot 1972.

Le Tissier, Jackie, *Food Combining for Health*,
     Northamptonshire: Thorson's 1992.

Mansfield, Dr Peter and Monro, Dr Jean, *Chemical
     Children*, London: Century 1987.

Martlew, Gillian and Silver, Shelly, *The Medicine Chest*,
     Northamptonshire: Thorson's 1988.

Mayes, Kathleen, *Brittle Bone and Osteoporosis — The
     Calcium Crisis*, London: Grapevine 1987.

Miller, Saul and Miller, Jo Anne, *Food for Thought*, New
     Jersey: Prentice Hall 1979.

Mindell, Earl, *The Vitamin Bible*, London: Arlington
     Books 1979.

Mindell, Dr Earl, *The Vitamin Bible for your Children*,
     London: Arlington Books 1981.

Nambudripad, Dr, *Say Goodbye to Illness*, California: Delta
     Publishing 1993.

Pekkanen, John, 'Seven Health Symptoms You Must Not
     Ignore', in *Reader's Digest*, London: Reader's Digest
     October 1992.

Permaculture Magazine, Hyden House, Little Hyden Lane, Clanfield, Hampshire: Permanent Publications.

Pfinter, A., *Composting, An Introduction to the Rational Use of Organic Waste*, Switzerland: Co-operative Migros, 1981.

Pitchford, Paul, *Healing with Whole Foods: Oriental Traditions and Modern Nutrition*, California: North Atlantic Books 1993.

Poesnecker, G. E., *Adrenal Syndrome, The Disease No Doctor Wants to Treat*, Pennsylvania: Humanitarian Publishing 1983.

Price, Dr Weston, *Nutrition and Physical Degeneration*, DDS Santa Monica, California, Price-Poltenger Foundation 1970.

Rapp, Doris J., *Allergies and your Family*, London: Sterling Publications 1981.

Rogers, Dr Sherry A., *Tired or Toxic?*, New York: Prestige 1990.

Sheinkin, Dr David, Schachter, Dr Michael and Hutton, Richard, *Food — Mind and Mood*, New York: Warner Books 1979.

Shreeve, Dr Caroline, *An Alternative Dictionary of Symptoms and Cures*, London: Random House 1995.

Shulman, Anne, *The Holistic Approach to Detoxification and Colon Care*, London: Green Library 1996.

Smith, Dr Lendon, *Feed your Kids Right*, New York: Dell Publishing 1979.

Trattler, Ross, *Better Health through Natural Healing: How to Get Well without Drugs or Surgery*, Northamptonshire: Thorson's 1987.

Vogel, Dr, *The Nature Doctor*, Edinburgh: Mainstream Publishing Co., 1990.

Wade, Carlson, *Helping your Health with Enzymes*, New York: Arco Publishing 1966.

Wade, Carlson, *Magic Minerals*, New York: Arco Publishing 1967.

Weeks, Nora, *The Medical Discoveries of Dr Bach*, Saffron Walden: C. W. Daniel 1940.

Weil, Dr Andrew, *Spontaneous Healing*, London: Little Brown 1995.

FURTHER READING

Chopra, Deepak, *Perfect Health*, London: Bantam, 1990.

Chopra, Deepak, *Quantum Healing*, London: Bantam, 1986.

Feist, Sr Theresa, *Spirituality and Holistic Living*, Dublin: Mercier Press 1990.

Henry Doubleday Research Association (HDRA), Monthly Publications, Bocking Braintree, Essex.

Hoffman, David, *New Holistic Herbal*, Dorset: Element Books 1983.

Lewis, Alan, *The Natural Athlete*, London: Century 1984.

Mumby, Dr Keith, *Complete Guide to Food Allergies*, London: Thorson's 1993.

Prevention Magazine, Hertfordshire: Rodale Press.

Scott, Julian, *Natural Medicine for Children*, London: Unwin Paperbacks 1990.

Sinha, Phulgenda, *Yogic Cure for Common Ailments*, New Delhi: Vision Books 1980.

Index